D0288330

101 WAYS

TO THE

BEST MEDICAL

CARE

Charlotte E. Thompson, M.D.

ISBN 0-7414-3327-3

Published by:

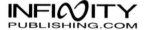
PUBLISHING.COM

1094 New DeHaven Street, Suite 100
West Conshohocken, PA 19428-2713
Info@buybooksontheweb.com
www.buybooksontheweb.com
Toll-free (877) BUY BOOK
Local Phone (610) 941-9999
Fax (610) 941-9959

Printed in the United States of America
Printed on Recycled Paper
Published July 2006

To
Jerry King
and
all those who
said this book
must be written

TABLE OF CONTENTS

INTRODUCTION

Jane and Roger were vacationing in a coastal village on the last day of a relaxing three-day weekend. Jane was lying in a lounge chair, enjoying the sun and the treasured time off. She reached back to make her chair go a little lower and felt searing pain. Her finger was caught in the chair. Roger jumped up to help and pulled Jane free. Her fingertip was gone and there was profuse bleeding. The couple knew no one in the small village and especially not a doctor. They were given directions to the local hospital, but found it to be small and crowded. What could Roger do to ensure his wife received the best possible medical care?

Knowing how to navigate the medical maze is daily becoming more important. *Your life can depend on it.* You, not your doctor, have the ultimate responsibility for your health.

Few doctors now have a direct relationship with their patients. Instead, there are layers of staff people and administrators. Patients are "consumers" of health care that has been taken over by corporations.

Some wonderful physicians still practice, but they are greatly limited in their ability to be your advocates. Instead, they are under constant pressure to limit care, the time they spend with patients, and cost. New government regulations, such as privacy rules and complex billing, have created havoc and dramatically increased a physician's paper work.

The goal in *101 Ways To The Best Medical Care* is to help individuals learn how to obtain the best possible medical care, to recognize quality care, as well as substandard care. It is too easy to be influenced by glitzy HMO and insurance company marketing. Accepting inadequate medical care can cause irreparable harm to you and your loved ones. Your choice of doctors, an HMO, or insurance company could mean the difference between good health, a lifetime of suffering, or even death.

I hope this book will help readers learn how to navigate the medical maze, so they will be in charge and get the best possible medical care.

CHAPTER ONE

General Advice

"The health care system in the United States is broken". We hear this daily from patients, doctors, and even legislators. Fifty percent of our nation's bankruptcies are said to be caused by medical bills. Forty-six million people in the U.S. are without health coverage. We are the richest nation in the world, so how can this be? Managed care has become "mangled care". Horror studies abound with vivid descriptions of greedy administrators of HMOs and insurance companies, disinterested doctors, and excessive drug company profits. There are still some wonderful, caring physicians, but they have to work harder and harder to keep up with the ever increasing paperwork and their decreasing incomes. Insurance premiums keep rising, as CEOs and administrators want to make more and more money. *One man with a five-figure income said, "Pretty soon all I'll be working for is to pay my family's medical insurance."* Until there is a national uproar demanding a change in health care, each of us must learn how to work with the present cumbersome and grossly inadequate medical system.

Rules to Live By

1. **Always insist on the best medical care possible. It could be a matter of life and death.**

   Roger, Jane's husband, was desperate to get help for his wife. He waited outside the emergency room and when someone went in who looked like a doctor, he stopped the individual and pled his case. His fighting spirit got his wife faster care and may have saved her hand.

No patient should have to fight to get good medical care, but that is what is happening in the U.S. Ideally, a patient would have a patient advocate, a physician, or attorney to help fight HMOs, insurance companies, and hospitals to get needed medical care. Now it is the responsibility of each of us to educate ourselves about ways to get the medical care we need. If you are very wealthy, you can pay private companies large sums of money to be your advocate. That seems unreal to me when part of my work as a physician has been to help patients and friends find the best medical care possible. To get this kind of medical care, my recommendations are the following:

Don't accept care from a non-physician, unless there is direct supervision by a doctor. Some medical offices allow untrained personnel to do procedures or tasks.

I was referred to an ophthalmologist to get a prescription for glasses. The young man who did the actual testing said he had no medical training, but was a high school graduate. The eye doctor came into the room after the untrained technician had done the examination and written the prescription. He smiled, was pleasant, signed the Rx, and went on his way. It turned out the prescription was completely wrong. (Yes, my insurance was billed the full amount for the eye doctor's time, not the low rate of the high school graduate who did the actual testing!) I tried two other ophthalmology offices and was told their doctors also had individuals without medical training do their examinations for glasses. Thus, I traveled 600 miles to see my previous, excellent eye doctor. He was amazed when he looked at the Rx given to me by the untrained technician. *The Rx had no relation to the one my tried-and-true ophthalmologist gave me.*

Sometimes you have to see multiple physicians before you find one who is interested in you and not the money your visit will bring. If you have signed up for care in an HMO, you are greatly restricted in your ability to find the best physicians. Thus, before a decision is made to sign away your rights with an HMO, careful investigation needs to be made about the physicians in the group. Do they use personnel without medical training to do procedures or examinations and what rights do you have to leave the HMO or appeal their decisions?

****

This true case history of a hard-working professional shows how a single illness can change your life unless good medical care is received.

A fifty-year-old single woman, Bernice, developed severe chest pain and shortness of breath. She was seen in the emergency room of the health plan facility and given an electrocardiogram (EKG), but was not hospitalized. Instead, she was sent home with medicine. The next day, she drove herself to see her health plan physician who told her she had an inflammation of the lining of the heart (pericarditis). She was not referred to a heart doctor (cardiologist) and hospitalization was not suggested. Again, she was sent home. With no close family or friends, the woman tried to care for herself, as best she could. She did survive, but paid dearly for her inadequate medical care by losing many months of work. She did not feel well for several years afterward.

If this patient had been hospitalized and received proper rest and care, the outcome could have been very different. Instead, she had to try to feed and care for herself when she had a potentially life-threatening heart disorder. If she had been hospitalized, as she should have been, health care aides could have been provided on discharge. This would have taken a prescription from her doctor. The physician would have had to ask the patient about her home situation and contact a discharge planner to make the necessary arrangements. This could have been done in five to ten minutes.

2. **Don't be your own physician.** Doctors are among the worst, in this regard. They often don't want to bother a colleague with their medical problems or those of family members. (Ego can also be involved.) There are occasions when a doctor has to prescribe for himself or herself, because it is impossible to find a physician willing, interested, or knowledgeable enough to provide the necessary care.

A doctor diagnosed his chest pain as indigestion and treated himself with Maalox and Tums. When he became cold and sweaty, his wife took charge and drove him to a nearby emergency room. Here he was found to have had a heart attack and was immediately hospitalized.

Many people these days are so fed up with the current medical system that they treat themselves with herbal or over-the-counter medicines (OTC) or consult individuals who claim to have answers for their medical problems. Alternative medicine can frequently lessen symptoms. Acupuncture performed by a licensed, experienced individual may help some ailments. However, the individual's credentials should be carefully investigated before any treatment is allowed. There are M.D.s, who are also acupuncturists, so they may be especially good. Massage can also relieve stress and muscle aches. My excellent internist once gave me the card of a massage therapist he had seen. She provided some stress relief at a time when I very much needed it.

One doctor kept a big bottle of penicillin in the linen closet. Whenever anyone in the family felt ill, he or she took a few pills. When one of the kids told me this, I said to the parents, "Either get rid of the penicillin bottle or find a new doctor." The pills were flushed down the toilet.

3. **You know your own body better than anyone else and how your body reacts to different medications and situations.** If a doctor won't listen, a serious problem could develop. Some individuals have bad reactions to "normal" doses of medicines. Doses of medications are listed in the *Physicians Desk Reference* (PDR), which is available in most libraries, Doses are given for both adults and children and every physician is sent this reference book yearly. However, no two patients are the same and the dose for one may not be appropriate for another.

A physician, who was quite small, was to have a surgical procedure and told the anesthesiologist prior to surgery that she didn't need large or adult doses of medicine. The doctor either didn't listen or discounted what the woman said. He gave her an adult dose of atropine prior to her surgery, which caused a severe reaction. (Atropine is a drug that reduces secretions but can cause a rapid heart rate and an extremely dry mouth.) The patient suffered unnecessarily. She was in no great danger, but had a very unpleasant time because the anesthesiologist paid no attention to what he was told.

4. If a doctor or other health care professional says nothing is wrong with you and you know there is, keep looking for answers until you find them. Be sure however, that you have a legitimate complaint, because there are patients who thrive on doctors' attention and seek help unnecessarily.

A teenager fell and hurt her wrist and hand. Her father and grandfather, both physicians, thought she had just bruised her hand or sprained it. The girl kept insisting something was broken. To humor her, the father had an X-ray taken of her wrist and hand. A small fracture of one of the bones of the wrist was found and a cast was put on the girl's hand. She was glad she had insisted something was wrong.

****

A teacher tripped over a stool and hurt her ankle. She drove to the urgent care center of her health plan and said she wouldn't leave until an X-ray was taken. No fracture was seen, so an Ace bandage was wrapped around her ankle and she was sent home. When the pain became worse, the woman called the doctor parent of one of her students. He called the urgent care center and the nurse pulled the teacher's X-rays. "I think I see a fracture of one of the small foot bones", she said. The teacher returned to the urgent care center and a different doctor agreed there was a fracture. He put a cast on the woman's leg for support and her foot felt much better, as soon as the cast was in place. The teacher was delighted she had insisted there was a problem.

5. Don't let doctors or their office staffs intimidate you. If you do, it will be difficult to get the best care. If you find it hard or impossible to stand up for yourself, take a family member or good friend with you who is not intimidated by medical people. There will always be people who thrive on keeping others under their control. Learning how to handle yourself with individuals like this takes experience and a stiff backbone. Once you learn how to handle them, either with honey or your "big voice", you will have accomplished a major goal. No one should ever make you feel ignorant or inadequate.

****

An extremely competent, successful professional said she "turned into a jellyfish in the doctor's office". Because of this, she received very inadequate care. After months of poor health, her daughters took charge, went with her to the appointments, and insisted she change physicians.

****

In contrast to the professional woman, a seventeen-year old college student, Jana, made an appointment to see a doctor at the student health service because of a respiratory infection. When she was called in to the examining rooms, the nurse said, "You are seeing Dr. Y." "No," said the college freshman, "I don't know anything about Dr. Y. I have an appointment with Dr. X and that is who I want to see. My parents are both doctors and she is the one they told me to see." The nurse took a deep breath and took Jana to see Dr. X!

******

6. **Be willing to pay for the best medical care you can afford.** Due to HMO and insurance company restrictions, many people don't look outside their health plan for the best physicians. Even many extremely wealthy people

feel medical care should cost little or nothing. They often pay large amounts for luxuries but skimp on money for medical services. Then they complain about the quality of care received. *Even individuals with limited income need to put money aside regularly for medical care.* Good medical care is far more important than a large, expensive TV set. You usually get what you pay for.

A fifty-five-year-old professional woman always bought expensive designer clothes. She believed she needed these to look her best. To save money, she joined an HMO. When medical problems developed, the specialists she wanted to see were not on the HMO's list of doctors. The woman resented having to pay for outside specialists and realized what a bad mistake she had made by joining an HMO. However, she didn't change her health plan and continued spending money on clothes rather than paying for health insurance that would allow her to choose her own doctors. She could have avoided this risk by choosing a better health care plan and a higher deductible. Thus, she would have saved money on a monthly basis, but would have had better care in the event of a major accident or illness.

****

If you pay for your own medical care and choose a special physician who does not accept HMO or insurance company restrictions, payment issues should be discussed prior to or on your first visit. Then, there will be no surprises. It is extremely important when you see these special physicians, to pay your bills promptly and on time. *Not all doctors are wealthy.* The majority make far less than CEOs of insurance companies, HMOs, and corporation executives. Pediatricians are at the bottom of the medical income scale. The CEOs are taking home millions of dollars in annual pay, whereas many outstanding doctors have to be extremely careful about how they spend their hard-earned money.

Other physicians are refusing to be in traditional HMOs and are asking patients to pay either a one-time "access" fee to use their services or to pay a monthly retainer fee. There is some question that this is legal and the American Medical Association (AMA) has set up some guidelines for these "*boutique*" or "*concierge*" practices. The up-front charge may be several thousand dollars, which the doctors say makes it possible for them to give better care to a small number of patients. Insurance and Medicare are usually not billed and there is a question if Medicare will pay expensive charges: CT scans, MRIs, surgeries, or hospitalizations. A national organization, MDVIP, is supporting boutique or concierge practices.

The doctors in these expensive practices say they can offer more preventive care, decrease waiting time, and be immediately available for care. This may be fine for the affluent patients, who can afford their care. Restricting care to those few who can pay for it raises ethical and moral issues. I believe that the practice of medicine should not be about money but about offering the best possible care to patients of all incomes.

7. **Do some preparation before you go for an appointment to a doctor's office, particularly if medical personnel intimidate you.** Writing down your questions before a visit is a good idea. Think through what you want to say and what you want to find out. *Expect that your questions will be answered.* If the questions bother a doctor, change doctors. If you are uncomfortable about asking questions, take along a family member or friend to the doctor's appointment. (At times, we all need an advocate who can speak up on our behalf.)

Juanita went to see her doctor for the annual check-up following a mastectomy. Because the cancer was removed, the doctor did an examination and was about to walk quickly out the examining room door. Juanita politely, but firmly, reminded him that she came a long distance and only saw him once a year. She said she had several questions. To the doctor's credit, he realized that he had been quite rushed. So he sat down and patiently answered Juanita's questions. At the next year's visit, the doctor knew there would be questions and didn't rush out the door.

If you are taking several medications, take along a list with the names and dosages. (You can also take the bottles, but this is cumbersome.) If you expect to see more than one doctor, make several copies of your list. It's important to note any allergies to medications or other things. Be sure and update the list as needed.

Take along the names, addresses, and telephone numbers of family members that you would give permission for medical personnel to contact. This can be extremely important, particularly if you have a serious medical condition.

Make a list of medical procedures and surgeries you have had and note the dates, where the procedures were done, and the names of the doctors. If you are to have an anesthetic and have had reactions to anesthetics in the past or if someone in your family has a neuromuscular disorder, this is important information for a doctor to know. A condition called "Malignant Hyperthermia" is associated with some muscle diseases. If a patient has Malignant Hyperthermia, a serious or fatal reaction can occur during surgery, when certain anesthetic agents are used. This is preventable if an anesthesiologist is warned ahead of time.

Take notes if your doctor is discussing something important. *Tape-recording the conversation is probably not going to be welcome.* If you don't understand something, ask for and insist on an explanation in nonmedical language. Also, ask the doctor to write down any instructions you need and ask that prescriptions be printed on a separate piece of paper, so you can check the names of the drugs against what you receive from a pharmacy. When you get home and need to ask another question, call back, and leave a message for the doctor. If your call has not been returned, call again the next day.

Even the best doctors are not always clear. One medically astute patient, Connie, was given an Rx for "biweekly medication" by her excellent physician. Because Connie was paid biweekly, she thought she was supposed to take the prescription every other week, just like she received her paycheck. Several months later, she found out that the doctor meant she should take the medicine twice a week. In this situation, Connie didn't suffer any serious consequences, but she did not get the full benefit of the medicine. Misunderstanding about another type of medication, such as heart or cholesterol pills, could have been quite harmful.

CHAPTER TWO

Finding Good Doctors

Finding the best general doctor and needed specialists is critical to good health. Many wonderful, caring doctors still practice, although many older doctors are leaving practice because of new regulations and overwhelming paperwork.

General rules about finding the best doctors are:

8. **Calling your local medical society for doctors' names or looking in the Yellow Pages can be harmful to your health.** The staff at your local medical society is not allowed by law to give details about a physician. They may only disclose a physician's address, telephone number, and information regarding a specialty, if there is one. The best way to find out about a doctor is to ask other doctors or friends who have had experience with the physician. A few doctors are willing to be interviewed, such as the physician who will deliver your baby. Some doctors have Web sites. Other doctors advertise widely, but a large advertising budget is not necessarily an indication of a good doctor.

The list of the "Best Doctors in the United States" is not one I would recommend. It is often a list of the most popular doctors or those who get along well with their peers. A less social physician may be the one you want to see. Patients do not compile this list. Instead, it is put together by suggestions from other physicians.

If you are pregnant and want to find a pediatrician or family doctor for your newborn, your obstetrician should be able to recommend one or two good ones. With this recommendation, try to make an appointment to see if the doctor is someone you relate to and is on the staff of a hospital near you. While you are in the doctor's office, be sure you are comfortable with the office staff and that the office is clean and professional. It is important to check the hours and days that the office is open and to find out with which doctors the physician trades weekend and night calls. The doctor you have chosen may trade calls with someone you would not want to care for your baby.

9. **Networking with friends and family members will pay off, if you are looking for a new doctor or specialist.** If you find good doctors, spread the word among your neighbors, family, and friends. Good doctors may stay in practice longer knowing they are appreciated. We need to keep as many good ones as possible.

10. **Asking a doctor friend or his or her staff for a referral to another doctor may give good results.** However, beware of the doctors who are not likely to say anything negative about another doctor. Be careful too, that the doctor you are asking about is not the next-door neighbor, health club friend, or golf buddy of the physician to whom you are speaking. Social doctors may not be the ones you want to see, particularly if they spend a lot of time socializing at cocktail parties and drink even when they are on call.

> A single, professional woman moved across country to accept a position in a large corporation. One of her first priorities was to find a good doctor and dentist. Her mother was still in touch with a college friend who was married to a doctor in the city. With this doctor's recommendations, the young woman found

an excellent doctor, dentist, and other specialists as needed.

If you are new to a city and don't have connections, I would ask people at work, neighbors, and the doctors you had in another city. They may have one or more good referrals for you.

It is possible now to check a state medical society's Web site to see if a physician has had malpractice lawsuits filed against him or her. Remember, however, that some good physicians settle lawsuits at the suggestion of their insurance companies to avoid the time and stress involved in going to court. Because there are many lawsuit-happy individuals in the country today and some hungry lawyers, frivolous lawsuits do occur. There are lawsuits that should be filed when a patient has been harmed by a physician's carelessness or incompetence. Unfortunately, it takes some medical boards far too long to revoke licenses of incompetent physicians.

Boutique or Concierge Doctors

Some doctors are now restricting their practices to the patients who will pay a yearly fee from $1500 to as much as $20,000. For this, the doctors say they will be on-call twenty-four hours a day, seven days a week. They restrict their practice to 400 to 600 patients. Not only do they ask for the up-front fee, but some bill insurance companies and Medicare. Thus, this type of practice is for affluent individuals or those who have multiple medical problems and can afford the yearly fee.

Some problems that can occur are if the boutique doctor decides to stop practicing before the end of the year or if there are problems with the care. When either of these occurs, a patient needs to call the state attorney general's office. However, these offices are usually so overloaded that action may not be taken.

Health Professionals You May Encounter

Allergist: A physician with specialized training in the treatment of allergies in adults or children.

Anesthesiologist: An M.D. with several years of additional training giving anesthetics for surgical procedures. Some specialize in pain treatment.

Audiologist: A health professional, not a physician, with training in detecting and aiding those with hearing loss.

Cardiologist: A physician with specific training in diseases of the heart. Pediatric cardiologists have training in children's heart disorders. These doctors are not surgeons.

Dermatologist: A doctor with special training in diseases of the skin. There are pediatric dermatologists with training in skin diseases of children.

Dietitian: An individual with special training in diets and specific nutritional needs of the body. Dietitians are generally connected with hospitals, but some work independently.

Endocrinologist: A medical doctor with special training in treating endocrine diseases of children and adults. Endocrine glands are those concerned with hormones such as insulin, which relates to diabetes, and the production of thyroid hormones, which relate to growth and many other important functions of the body.

Family Practitioner: A physician who has had training in many specialties and sees both children and adult. He or she has often had more years of training than a general practitioner.

Gastroenterologist: A medical doctor with additional training in diseases of the gastrointestinal tract. Pediatric gastroenterologists are usually found in large cities or connected with children's hospitals.

General Practitioner: A physician who treats both children and adults. These doctors are not required to have specialized training.

Geriatrician: A medical doctor with training in internal medicine who cares for elderly individuals.

Geneticist: A physician who may have pediatric training and additional genetic training. There are genetic counselors, who may be nurses or other paramedical people.(*When a genetic condition in suspected, it is important to establish the diagnosis with certainty before seeking a genetic counselor, because counseling is difficult to give unless the exact type of disorder is known.*)

Gynecologist: A physician who specializes in treatment of problems with women's reproductive organs.

Hematologist: A medical doctor who may have either pediatric or internal medicine backgrounds. Hematologists treat disorders of the blood. Pediatric hematologists treat children with leukemia, anemia, sickle-cell disease, and any blood-related problems.

Internist: A medical doctor with additional training in adult disorders. Many internists have subspecialty training in gastroenterology, (diseases of the stomach and intestines), rheumatology, (diseases of the joints and related disorders). They generally see adults, but some see teenagers.

Immunologist: A medical doctor with special training in disorders of the immune system. The immune system is responsible for how our bodies react to foreign substances, viruses or bacteria.

Neonatologist: A pediatrician with additional training in the care of premature and newborn babies. They work in hospital nurseries.

Nephrologist: A physician who specializes in diseases of the kidneys.

Neurologist: A medical doctor with pediatric or adult training in disorders of the brain and nervous system.

Neuromuscular Specialist: These are physicians with specialized training in neuromuscular diseases of children and adults.

Nurse Practitioner: A registered nurse with additional training, allowing him or her to do certain examinations and procedures that registered nurses are not licensed to do.

Obstetrician: A physician who sees women during pregnancy and is responsible for delivery and immediate postpartum care. Obstetricians are also trained in gynecology, so they can provide ongoing care involving the female reproductive system.

Occupational Therapist: **(O.T.)** An individual with specific training in the function of the musculoskeletal system, particularly the upper extremities. Occupational therapists are involved in the developmental problems of children and also concerned with activities of daily living, such as dressing and eating, upper extremity strength, and how to adapt the environment to make it more workable for a disabled person.

Oncologist: A medical doctor who treats patients with tumors, both benign and malignant (cancers). Pediatric oncologists have had special training in caring for children's cancers.

Ophthalmologist: A medical doctor with several years of additional training in examining and treating disorders of the eyes. An ophthalmologist is a licensed surgeon and does eye surgery.

Optometrist: A doctor of optometry does not have a medical degree and is not licensed to issue or prescribe drugs. Optometrists can prescribe glasses, eye exercises, and contact lenses.

Orthopedic Surgeon: A physician with several years of postgraduate training in disorders of bones and joints. The orthopedist performs surgical procedures on the back and extremities. There are subspecialties of orthopedics: hand surgery, back surgery, and children's orthopedics.

Osteopath: An individual who has graduated from a school of osteopathy. Some states allow osteopaths to qualify for an M.D. degree. Their scope of treatment varies according to the school from which they graduated, but many are licensed to do almost the same things medical doctors do.

Otolaryngologist: A medical doctor with additional training in treating diseases of the ears, nose, and throat. There are some who see only ear problems. Some see children; others see both children and adults.

Pathologist: A medical doctor who is trained to make diagnoses by looking at microscopic sections and studying tumors or tissues that have been surgically removed.

Pediatrician: An M.D. with additional training in normal childhood development and the treatment of childhood diseases.

Pediatric Allergist: An allergist who treats children with allergic problems.

Pediatric Cardiologist: A cardiologist who specializes in children's heart problems.

Pediatric Dermatologist: A dermatologist who specializes in children's skin diseases.

Pediatric Endocrinologist: An endocrinologist who has special training in endocrine disorders of childhood.

Pediatric Neurologist: A neurologist who treats seizures and other childhood disorders of the brain and spinal cord.

Pediatric Orthopedist: An orthopedic surgeon who treats children's diseases of the bones and joints.

Pediatric Rheumatologist: A rheumatologist who treats rheumatoid arthritis in children and similar disorders.

Pharmacist: A drug information specialist. All practicing pharmacists are registered (R.Ph.'s) by their particular state board of pharmacy. All pharmacy schools now issue Doctor of Pharmacy degrees (Pharm.D.) and most graduates participate in a host of clinical residency programs in both inpatient (hospital) and outpatient (ambulatory care) settings.

Physiatrist: A medical doctor with additional training in rehabilitation or nonsurgical treatment of post-accident victims, back injuries, polio, and neuromuscular diseases.

Physical Therapist: (P.T.) An individual with training in the function of joints and muscles. Physical therapists evaluate and treat children and adults who have problems of the musculoskeletal system. They do this by teaching strengthening exercises, massage, or working with specific equipment to help strengthen muscles.

A doctor's Rx is usually required for them to give therapy. There are a few states that allow "Direct access" care. For this, you don't need a doctor's Rx, but you pay the costs, not an insurance company.

Physical Therapy Assistant: Someone who is licensed to do everything except evaluate a patient. They have had some physical therapy training.

Physical Therapy Technician: These individuals are not licensed and are trained on the job. Some training is available in different states.

Physical Therapy Aide: This individual may have no medical training but is trained by the therapists.

Plastic Surgeon: A surgeon with additional training in repair of facial problems or cosmetic surgery.

Podiatrist: A health professional who has graduated from a four-year college of podiatry. They specialize in the care of foot and leg problems. They are trained to do surgical procedures of problems below the knees. They are doctors of podiatry.

Pulmonologist: An M.D. with additional training in diseases of the lungs. There are both adult and children's pulmonologists.

Psychiatrist: A medical doctor who has had additional training in mental and emotional disorders. There are pediatric psychiatrists with a background in childhood disorders and adult psychiatrists. Some psychiatrists see patients just in hospitals; others practice only outpatient psychiatry.

Psychologist: An individual who has either a masters degree (M.A.) or a doctorate (Ph.D.) in psychology. Psychologists have had variable kinds of training in working with children and adults. Some do testing and therapy, others do just therapy. There are many different schools of psychology, as well as specialties.

Radiologist: A radiologist is a medical doctor who has had additional training in diagnosing conditions by X-ray, CAT scan, and MRI. Many radiologists do therapy on cancer patients.

Registered Nurse: An individual who has had nursing school training and works under the supervision of a physician. Now many nurses get additional training so they can do other types of procedures or examinations.

Rheumatologist: A physician who treats either children or adults. Rheumatologists have additional training, beyond pediatrics or internal medicine, in diseases involving the joints, for example, juvenile rheumatoid arthritis, and collagen or connective tissue diseases, as lupus erythematosus.

Social Worker: An individual with special training in counseling and finding resources for children and adults. Social workers have either a medical social worker (M.S.W.) or licensed clinical social worker (L.C.S.W.) degree.

Speech Pathologist: A professional with post-graduate training in diagnosing and treating speech and language disorders.

Urologist: A surgeon with specialized training in treating disorders and diseases of the urinary tract and kidneys. There are both pediatric and adult specialists.

CHAPTER THREE

Finding a Different Doctor

It is not difficult to change from one physician to another. A general physician or internist should be someone who respects your opinions, is caring, concerned, and not always rushed. Sometimes it may be necessary to change doctors several different times until you find just the right one.

11. **If you are not satisfied with a physician by the end of your first visit, change doctors!** No doctor should make you feel uncomfortable about asking questions, rush out of the room to answer multiple telephone calls, or spend very few minutes with you. Dictating in your presence is not professional and is something I would not accept. Medicine is much more than a quick examination. It is getting to know your patient and a physician can not do this in a few minutes. Taking a good history is an art and something that is learned by experience. *A good doctor sits down to talk with you.*

   A forty-five-year-old, single, professional woman had just moved to a big city and was referred to an internist. He had a good reputation, but as he did a physical examination, he seemed more interested in the woman's marital status than her health. As she was dressing after the examination, the doctor asked her for a date! She quickly said "Thank you, but I have a long time liaison with a man." The woman left as quickly as she could and immediately started looking for another physician. She found a great one after a search.

12. If a physician doesn't listen to your concerns or answer your questions, insist he or she does or change!

A grandmother, who was a practicing physician, took her grandson to see the Chief of Dermatology at a Children's Hospital, because of the child's severe eczema. When a young doctor-in-training started to do the examination, the grandmother said the appointment was with the staff doctor and they would wait for him. The dermatologist finally arrived and was very arrogant. After five minutes and a most inadequate examination, he started to leave. The grandmother said, "Excuse me, I have several questions." "Oh", he said, "I have to answer a phone call." The questions were never answered and the grandmother and her grandson left, knowing the visit had been a waste of time. Instead, they went to another city and saw a dermatologist who had been in medical school with the grandmother. He spent considerable time with the boy and did a thorough examination. When they left the twelve-year-old said, *"He's a real doctor. I've never had one like that before!"* (The boy had been seen by two other dermatologists in his hometown, in addition to the pediatric dermatologist.)

One woman told me she defines a "real" doctor as one who sits down to talk with you. Sitting takes extra time and means he or she probably won't rush immediately out of the room.

13. If your primary physician doesn't take a complete history or do a thorough physical examination, when that is what you expected, *change physicians!* An examination may take two or three visits before it is complete. A family history is also important to know about special family illnesses or problems, anesthetic

reactions, or diseases that occur frequently in members of the extended family.

An older woman saw a new physician because her previous physician had sold his practice. After two visits, the doctor still had not taken a history or done a physical examination. Instead, she kept ordering batteries of tests. The patient wasn't assertive enough to ask what the tests were for. Her sons, daughters, and doctor friends insisted she change doctors. They couldn't understand why a doctor would keep ordering blood tests when she hadn't examined the woman. (The answer is that it takes longer to do a good history and physical than to check a lab slip and send the patient out the door.)

14. **If you need to speak with a physician and are never allowed to do so, change doctors!** In most offices these days, secretaries, aides, or nurses answer the phone calls. Often just a machine answers. One woman said the office phone of her pediatrician was the only doctor's office phone that she had found answered by a human! Routine phone calls are not always *routine.* If you need to speak with your doctor, you may have to become assertive to get past the front office staff. Your call may not be returned until later in the day, but should be returned. If you make multiple, unnecessary calls, it is understandable that your call will not be returned by the physician.

A mother called my office after hours saying her child, Joey, had fallen on something sharp and cut his mouth. Fortunately, I was able to answer the call immediately and said I wanted to see Joey right away even though his mother was resistant. It took a while for the mother to come to the office, but when she did, everyone was very glad. Joey had fallen on a sharp object, and I saw a large hole in the roof of his mouth. Immediate surgery was needed.

****

If you need to speak with a physician after hours and are told he or she is on call but doesn't have a cell phone or pager that is unacceptable. Any physician who is on-call should be available.

> A physician called a doctor in another state about his brother-in-law. Paramedics had had to be called early in the morning because the brother-in-law had fallen. The doctor's answering service said the doctor did not carry a cell phone or pager, and all they could do was leave a message in his office. Upon calling the office as soon as it opened, the man was told that the doctor didn't come in until 2:00 p.m. to see patients and they had no way to reach him. The brother-in-law's doctor finally called back a week later despite more phone calls and even a letter!

The physician had to use some strong words to convince his brother-in-law to change doctors. The probable incentive for changing came when the state medical board's Web site revealed the brother-in-law's doctor had been involved in a major lawsuit because a patient died without adequate care.

15. **To change to a different doctor, a written request should be faxed or mailed to your doctor asking that a copy or summary of your medical records be sent to the new physician.** It is wise to check with the new doctor's secretary after two or three weeks to be sure your records have been received and are adequate. Medical records are the property of the attending doctor, though some patients feel they should be given the entire record, if they change physicians. The armed services allowed

this in the past, but no longer do so. Doctors in private practice keep records for their own information and may record personal observations and notes that are not for a patient's eyes. Doctors should always provide summaries, copies of lab, and X-ray reports.

A ten-year-old boy was followed for several months by his pediatrician for an enlarged gland (lymph node) under his jaw. The pediatrician didn't seem concerned, but the parents decided it was time to get a second opinion and perhaps change doctors. They consulted another pediatrician who did a complete examination. In looking at his weight and asking about previous weights, she was concerned that there had been some weight loss. The boy was still eating well and seemed o.k. otherwise. The doctor ordered some blood work and found that two of the tests were abnormal. The physician told the parents she wanted their son to be seen by a child's cancer specialist and that the node should be removed. The parents immediately took their son to the specialist. The node was removed, and the boy was found to have Hodgkin's disease. The parents were angry that their previous doctor had not sent them to a specialist and had seemed so unconcerned about the node. They immediately faxed a request for the records to be sent to the new pediatrician.

One woman, Mrs. O, had been referred to a physician but decided to change after her third visit. Each time the doctor was with her in the examining room, there would be a knock on the door after five to ten minutes and one of the staff would say," Doctor, there's an important call for you." The third time this occurred, the woman became angry said, "Please tell the caller that the doctor is with Mrs. O and can not be disturbed."

****

An eighty-year-old man, with multiple health problems, was told he had diabetes. This was based on one blood glucose test of 131. (The normal range is 60-100). No other tests were done. Instead, he was sent to a class to learn about diabetes and given a blood sugar measuring instrument. No instructions about diet or medicine were given. Fortunately, the man's nephew was a physician. He was appalled that a diagnosis of diabetes was made on a single blood sugar test. He insisted that a diabetes specialist be consulted, either an internist specializing in diabetes or an endocrinologist. The uncle agreed and was subsequently found to have borderline diabetes. The man was given medication and a diet and decided it was finally time to change physicians. This was something his family had urged for several years.

****

A forty-year-old-woman, in good health, saw her gynecologist for a routine checkup and Pap smear. After the doctor examined her, he said, "You need a D & C." (A scraping of the lining of the uterus). "Why", asked the woman? The doctor could not give her a good answer, so the patient sought a second opinion. The second doctor said she saw no reason for the D & C and said the Pap smear was negative. Later, the woman discovered that the first gynecologist did routine D & Cs, on every patient at age forty! She also found out that the doctor had recently purchased a new expensive car, a large cabin cruiser, and was building a new house.

CHAPTER FOUR

Getting the Best Care

There are some general rules about getting the best medical care. Knowing how to work within the present medical system and being in charge of your own health takes time and energy. It is important to know as much as possible about today's medicine.

16. Educate yourself about medical terms.

If you don't understand a term or name that a health professional uses, ask the individual to explain the term to you in lay language. Often physicians and other medical personnel think they are using nonmedical terms when they are not. No patient should be embarrassed about saying, "Please explain that term, I'm not sure what it means."

17. Educate yourself about types of specialists and what you should expect from each.

It is wise to remember that just because a physician has initials after his or her name or has had training in an excellent medical school, he or she may not be the best. Some physicians start out giving excellent care, but, after awhile, they become sloppy or more interested in making money rather than taking care of patients. Some, too, develop drug or alcohol problems that begin to take their toll.

A physician was giving advice on a national television program. When he was asked what should be done if you have the 'flu', he replied, "You should take Tylenol and drink lots of fluids." The doctor should have added, "Remember the 'flu' may not be the 'flu'. You could have pneumonia and antibiotics might be necessary. It would be better to call your doctor rather than assuming what you have is the 'flu'. Kids should always be checked, if they seem quite ill. They could have a strep throat, ear infections, meningitis, or something else that needs immediate treatment. Elderly individuals are particularly at risk during flu season, and many die each year with untreated pneumonia."

18. Learn what titles or initials mean

M.D.- Medical doctor-An individual who has had four years training in an accredited medical school. To be awarded an M.D., specific tests must be passed. Before practicing, an additional training period or internship is required. To specialize in a branch of medicine, three or more years of additional training or residency are required and tests, called boards, must be passed.

D.O.- Osteopath- An individual who graduated from a four-year school of osteopathy. Some states allow D.O.s to receive a doctor of medicine degree, if tests are taken and passed. The D.O. can then apply to a program for additional training or residency in a medical school to complete board requirements in a specific field of medicine.

Ph.D.- Doctor of philosophy- These individuals may teach in a college or university, or may be licensed psychologists.

Board Certified - Specific tests in a specialty have been passed after the required training in a particular field of medicine has been completed.

Board Eligible- Specialized training has been received, but board examinations have not been taken or passed.

D.C.- Doctor of Chiropractic-(Chiropractor)-These individuals specialize in joint and spinal alignment.

P.A.- Physician's Assistant-To be certified as a P.A., the individual must have had a training course and pass certain tests. They are not nurses.

N.P.- Nurse Practitioner-Is a registered nurse with additional training of variable length.

R.N.- Registered Nurse- May have a college degree, but this is not necessary for some nursing programs.

A.P.R.N. - Registered nurses with additional education. Many have a master's degree. The group includes: certified nurse practitioner, certified nurse-mid-wife, and certified nurse anesthetist.

L.P.N. or **L.V.N.**- Licensed Practical Nurse or Licensed Vocational Nurse. They must have a high school education, plus a twelve to fourteen month course on basic nursing care. A licensing exam must be passed.

C.N.A.- Certified Nursing Assistant. These individuals receive training to provide non-medical care: bathing, dressing, and helping with bathroom needs.

O.D.- Optometrist-Can prescribe glasses, but not do surgery. The individual must have graduated from an accredited school of optometry.

O.T.- Optician-May have no training or just a few weeks in an eye doctor's office.

D.D.S.- Dentist-There are different types of dentists. Some have special training in diseases of the gum (peridontist) and others in straightening teeth (orthodontist).

M.F.C.C.- Marriage and Family Therapist-These individuals have postgraduate training in counseling and can work in clinics or have their own private practice.

M.F.T. - Marriage and Family Therapist-These are the new initials for an M.F.C.C.

L.C.S.W.- Licensed Clinical Social Worker-These professionals have additional training beyond their degree in social work. They are licensed to see patients without the supervision of a physician.

M.S.W.- Medical Social Worker-These are individuals who have graduated from an accredited school of social work. They find solutions for complex family and social problems and are experts at finding community resources for patients. They are attached to clinics or hospitals.

F.A.C.S.- Fellow of the American College of Surgeons-This means a surgeon has completed a prescribed course of training and passed specific board examinations.

F.A.A.P.- Fellow of the American Academy of Pediatrics

F. A.A.N.- Fellow of the American Academy of Neurology

F.A.C.O- Fellow of the American College of Otolaryngology

F.A.C.O.S.- Fellow of the American College of Orthopedic Surgeons

F.A.C.P.- Fellow of the American College of Physicians

F.A.P.A.- Fellow of the American Psychiatric Association

R.P.T.- Registered Physical Therapist (P.T.)-An individual with training in the structure and function of joints and muscles. They do evaluations and provide treatments for musculoskeletal problems. Specific prescriptions should be provided by an attending physician.

O.T.R.- Occupational Therapist (O.T.)-These are individuals who have training in the function and structure, particularly of the upper extremities. They teach activities of daily living (ADL) and work with children who have upper extremity problems or developmental delay.

19. **Getting to know your doctor's staff by name may help you get the best care. Being courteous and pleasant with all the staff will make you a patient who will be remembered.** Even though there may be staff members who are controlling or not friendly, try to win them over with pleasantness. If they are rude or unpleasant, then I would let the doctor know. Some physicians have a hard time firing staff members. Others may be unaware of how those in the outer office are treating their patients.

> One woman was extremely rude to the staff each time she came to the doctor's office, but always put on her best face for the physician. After a few visits, the doctor sent her a certified letter asking that she find medical care in another office.

20. **Paying your bills on time and not *bouncing* checks will make you a favorite.** According to many doctors, the patients who demand the most attention are the ones who are slow to pay their bills, have to receive constant reminders, or don't pay their bills at all. When patients do not pay their bills and are finally turned over to a collection agency, the return rate can be as low as twenty percent. It is easy to understand why good physicians join large groups because of their frustration about the patients who are demanding but don't pay their bills.

Some insurance companies send payments for the doctors directly to the patients. This should not happen. If you receive an insurance check that is a doctor's payment, it should be endorsed, signed over to the doctor, and sent to his or her office. Keeping the money is stealing from the doctor. Sometimes even the best patients are unaware the insurance money is not meant for them and the checks are not sent on to their doctors. It would be a good idea to make a copy of the check before you send it on, in case it is lost or stolen.

21. Keeping appointments and being on time will make you a favorite patient. Also, it is very discourteous to sit in the waiting room talking on a cell phone.

Try to use your cell phone only for urgent calls and move outside or to a corner, where you can not be overheard. I've been in offices where signs are posted saying, "Please step outside to use a cell phone", yet people are making and taking cell phone calls. They deliberately ignore the signs or chose not to see them. Using a cell phone in a medical office waiting room is not just discourteous, but cell phones can interrupt the functioning of pacemakers and other medical equipment.

22. If you make unusual demands on a physician's time or that of his or her office staff, you are less likely to receive good care. Making frequent unnecessary calls to the doctor or office staff will be remembered. If you have a real emergency, you might not get the quick action you need. Some patients are very "needy" and use doctor visits to fill their lonely days. Those who misuse their doctor's services are quickly identified and not as welcome as other patients.

23. If your doctor has provided excellent care, saying "thank you" or sending a thank you note or card will be appreciated. A Christmas or holiday thank you will be appreciated. (Some cookies or a small gift will be remembered).

> One special grandmother brought a cake each time she came to see me with her grandchild. Another woman brought warm Irish bread and butter. My staff and I always looked forward to these visits. We immediately would stop what we were doing, if this was possible, and take a five minute break to have coffee and a piece of these special treats.

24. There are doctors who have a wonderful bedside manner but have lost or never had adequate diagnostic skills. Run-of-the mill problems can often be resolved by more exercise, a better diet, or less stress. A physician who listens and cares may be all that is needed. However, if you have a major health problem, it is a different story. Don't be deceived by a great bedside manner that is not accompanied by good diagnostic skills.

> A seventy-eight-year-old woman began having dizzy spells and saw her general practitioner, who belonged to an HMO. The doctor didn't seem worried and said for the patient to get more rest. The woman's son, a dermatologist, was extremely worried about his mother and called the physician. The general practitioner asked the son what tests he would like to have done. This mystified the son because his specialty had nothing to do with dizziness in an elderly woman. He did suggest some tests, which the G.P. ordered. The tests were all negative but the mother continued having dizzy spells.

> The son did some research and found an internist in private practice who was strongly recommended. The son urged his mother to see this doctor. However, the

mother refused because she loved her G.P., who excelled in the art of medicine, but lacked greatly in diagnostic skills. Twelve days later, the mother had a stroke and died.

25. **Remember that doctors are human and get tired like everyone else. Try to be understanding if your doctor seems overworked.** If he or she is always tired, it might be time to look for a new physician because an overly tired doctor can make mistakes. Doctors-in-training in hospitals are usually overworked and overtired. If you are hospitalized, it is most important to have a family member or friend stay with you. Not only are the doctors tired and overworked but the ratio of R.N.s to patients is being severely cut by hospitals to save money. Many hospitals are using registry nurses, so benefits don't have to be paid to full-time staff. This does not allow continuity of care, which is extremely important for hospital patients. Some medically astute patients make certain that, if they have to have surgery, they schedule it early in the day when the doctor is fresh or on a day when he or she has a light schedule.

26. **If the medical appointment is for you, it is a good idea to leave your children with a baby-sitter or friend**. The doctor's staff is not licensed to run a child-care center. If you do take children to a doctor's office, be sure to take along some books or quiet toys. Be careful about taking messy snacks. Children should know they are expected not to yell or bang noisy toys.

> One excellent mother brought along a DVD player with a children's cartoon. Her four-year-old sat quietly watching the movie while I examined her sister. We all appreciated the mother's kindness in planning a quiet activity for her little girl.

Common Medical Terms

B.E.-Barium enema- an X-ray taken of the lower part of the bowel after a special enema preparation has been given.

B.I.D.-Instructions on a prescription indicating the medicine should be taken twice a day.

Biopsy-A piece of tissue removed from the body for the purpose of diagnosis. The tissue should be examined by a specialist. A muscle biopsy should always be done using a local anesthetic because of the possibility of Malignant Hyperthermia.

Collagen diseases-Included in this group are: rheumatoid arthritis, scleroderma, periarteritis nodosa, and lupus erythematosus. Rheumatologists are the specialists who should treat these disorders.

Cholesterol-A substance found in the blood and cells of the body. Two types are present: LDH is low-density lipoprotein, which can block arteries and HDL is high-density protein, which is believed to help protect arteries from blockage. Increased blood pressure (hypertension), heart attacks, and stroke can result from high cholesterol levels.

Colonoscopy-Direct visualization of the lower bowel performed under anesthetic.

CT scan -Special detailed X-ray study. The initials stand for computerized tomography.

DNR-Do not resuscitate.

EEG-(Electroencephalogram) Electrical recording of the brain waves.

EKG-(Electrocardiogram) Recording of electrical impulses from the heart.

EMG-(Electromyogram) Electrical impulses recorded from muscle.

Endocrine glands-Organs in the body that regulate various body functions: thyroid gland, pituitary, pancreas, adrenal glands, and parathyroid.

Exudate-A fluid or pus-containing substance that can be seen on tonsils with some sore throats or coming from a part of the body.

Fibromyalgia-Patients have diffuse muscle aches and pains. Regular exercise, decreasing stress, and injection of "trigger spots" can cause improvement. Trigger spots are painful points in muscles from which pain radiates. (President Kennedy was treated for fibromyalgia by his White House physician, Dr. Janet Travell.)

Flat plate-An X-ray of the abdomen taken without injection of any contrast substance.

False positive-Errors can occur when blood tests are performed. Also, certain conditions can occur which cause inaccurate results. For example, the CPK blood test, which can help check for muscle disease, can be unusually high if the patient has been very active prior to the test being taken. Blood sugars can be abnormally high, if a heavy intake of sugar containing foods has been ingested prior to the test.

False Negative-A blood test result found to be negative, when a repeat test is positive. This may be due to laboratory error or improper handling of the specimen.

Generic-This term is used for medications that are not licensed by a specific drug company or advertised and promoted by them. *If your doctor orders the generic brand of a drug, it will be much less expensive.* Every drug does not have a generic form and the drug companies try hard to keep drugs from having generic, cheaper forms.

H.S.-Instructions on a prescription indicating that the Rx should be taken at the hour of sleep.

Hypertrophy-Enlargement of an organ or extremity.

Hypothroid-Decreased function of the thyroid gland manifested by dry skin, constipation and lethargy.

Hyperthyroid-Increased function of the thyroid gland manifested by a rapid pulse, sweating and nervousness. Prominent eyes or exopthalmos can also occur.

I.M.-An injection given into the muscle (intramuscular).

I.V.-Fluid or a drug injected directly into the vein (intravenous).

I.C.U.-Intensive care unit.

I.V.P.-Kidney X-rays taken after an injection of a dye into a vein.

IPPB-Intermittent positive pressure breathing given to patients.

Irritable Bowel Syndrome-Cardinal signs are intermittent abdominal pain and loose bowel movements alternating with constipation.

Malignant Hyperthermia-A genetic disorder that occurs with the use of some anesthetics. It has a particular relationship to some of the muscle diseases. A high fever, tightness of the jaw and death can occur, if certain anesthetic agents are used.

Succinylcholine and halothane are two of the principal anesthetic agents to be avoided for patients with this disorder.

M.I.C.U.-Medical intensive care unit

MRI-(Magnetic resonance imaging)-A highly magnified X-ray study.

Nerve conduction times-Electrical impulses recorded from nerves.

N.I.C.U.-Newborn intensive care unit

NPO-Nothing by mouth after midnight. This is important prior to an anesthetic or some procedures and blood tests.

P.I.C.U.-Pediatric intensive care unit

Peritonitis-A serious infection in the abdomen- (A word ending in "itis" means infection).

Placebo-A pill containing nothing but a substance such as sugar. It is used in drug trials to see if a new drug is effective or acts the same as the fake one.

Sepsis-Infection in the blood stream, which can be extremely serious.

S.I.C.U.-Surgical intensive care unit

SMA-6, 12, 25-Special blood panel studies

STAT-This means a procedure, lab test, or drug must be done or given immediately.

T.I.D.-Instructions on a prescription that the medicine should be taken three times a day.

Upper GI - X-rays taken of the upper part of the gastrointestinal tract.

Vital signs - Blood pressure, pulse, respiratory rate, and temperature.

CHAPTER FIVE

HMO Rules and Regulations

HMOs or health maintenance organizations were first established in 1973 with the goal of limiting health care costs. Unfortunately, they have resulted in much poor care and many lawsuits. Gradually, now patients are finding that managed care is often "mangled care", as Dr. Robert LeBow states in his book, *Healthcare Meltdown*. To obtain even adequate care from an HMO, it is extremely important to understand how to navigate and frequently do battle with an HMO.

27. **If you are going to use an HMO for health care, becoming informed about how they function and learning their language is step number one.** HMOs have a language of their own. **Gatekeepers** are the physicians who decide which doctors you can and can not see and the tests, procedures, or surgeries you can or can not have. The gatekeeper could be your own physician or, most often, another one who knows nothing about you. Many decisions are made by office staff or administrators, *who do not have medical backgrounds.* Some companies hire R.N.s to make the decisions and these frequently overrule a physician's recommendation. This has led to many tragic outcomes and major lawsuits.

Other important terms and abbreviations are:

- **IPA**-Independent Practice Association -A group of physicians who practice in their own offices but who agree to abide by the payment plan and rules of an HMO. Each physician is paid a specified amount per patient in his or her care. The doctor receives this amount of money even though a patient needs no care. Individuals with chronic illness or multiple medical problems are not sought out as HMO members. Instead, an attempt is made to recruit a healthy group of patients.

- **PPO**-Preferred Provider Organization-Physicians who belong to a specific group. If you are a member of their group, you receive discounted fees. If you seek care from an "outside" physician, you will be responsible for a large part of his or her fee. In addition, you may find that a referral to an outside specialist will not be covered.

- **PCP**-Primary Care Provider-A physician who is responsible for your health care needs. He or she should make referrals to specialists as needed. Many are reluctant to make referrals as it can reduce their own pay. A "report card" is kept by many HMOs indicating how many referrals each physician makes. Referrals cost the HMO and physicians more and thus are greatly discouraged.

- **Capitation**-This is the amount of money an HMO pays a physician for every patient he or she is expected to see. The doctor makes more money, if the patients are not seen, tests are not requested, and referrals are not made to specialists.

- **Co-payment**-This is the amount of money you are asked to pay at each doctor's visit. The amount is variable according to the individual plan.

- **Preadmission Certification**-Hospital admissions for surgery or medical care have to be pre-approved by a representative from the HMO or insurance company. Nurses do this in most cases but your physician can insist on speaking with the Medical Director, if approval is not given. The doctor's office staff or the physician should arrange for a hospital admission.

  An orthopedic surgeon asked his secretary to call an insurance company in order to obtain approval for a ninety-three-year-old woman to have a total hip replacement. The secretary couldn't believe her ears when the answering clerk said, "This will be on a come-and-go basis in the emergency room, won't it?"

28. **If you decide to join an HMO for financial reasons, read all the rules and regulations very carefully before you enroll.** If you don't, there could be some bad surprises down the road. If you don't understand all of the language, call the HMO staff and try to get answers. Keep a record of what you are told and the name and telephone number of the individual to whom you have spoken. If you can't read the extremely fine print some of the HMOs use in their brochures, look through a magnifying glass. *It's important to read every word. Your life or that of a family member depends on it.*

The following are things you want to check carefully, before deciding to join an HMO:

- Are pre-existing conditions covered and how are these defined? Many HMOs and insurance companies will not provide coverage for pre-existing problems.

- Are hospitalizations covered and for how many days?

- Are you restricted as to which hospitals you can use?

- Is emergency care covered?

- Is ER care covered in a hospital not associated with the HMO or one that is out of state?

- Do you have a choice of doctors?

- Can you change doctors, if you are dissatisfied?

- Can you see a specialist, if you need to, who is not part of the HMO group of doctors?

- Can you see a specialist in the plan, if your primary doctor won't refer you?

- Is surgery covered and are there restrictions?

- Can one or more surgeries be covered?

- Are psychologists or psychiatrists covered for emotional problems or mental illness? If so, how many visits per month or year?

- Are prescriptions covered?

- Is drug addiction care covered?

- Is equipment covered: wheel chairs, walkers, lifts, commodes, hearing aids, braces, glasses, or respiratory equipment?

- Are cochlear implants covered?

- Is rehabilitative care covered and for how long?

- Is home health care covered and how many visits?

- Are routine tests covered such as:

Adults:

> Blood counts
>
> Urinalysis
>
> Chest x-rays
>
> Colonoscopy
>
> Mammograms
>
> Pap smears
>
> Cholesterol and other lab work

For children—are the following covered?

> Well baby exams
>
> Immunizations
>
> Yearly physicals
>
> TB skin tests
>
> Urinalysis
>
> Vision and hearing tests
>
> ER care
>
> Hospitalizations
>
> Surgeries
>
> Birth defects
>
> Specialists in HMO
>
> Specialists outside HMO
>
> Lab work
>
> X-rays

****

One family had a child with fixed joints. When medical care was required, the HMO didn't have specialists who could help her, but the HMO refused to pay for outside care. The specialist who saw the child called the medical director of the HMO and was told, "We are not responsible for the care of disabled children. That is up to the community or the school!" This family paid for the specialist themselves. Fortunately, the specialist greatly discounted her fee.

29. **If you plan to enroll in an HMO, do some research about the physicians you are permitted to see, before you enroll.** You may think you will be able to continue seeing your current physicians but then discover they are not part of the HMO group. If the HMO does not have specialists for one or more of your medical problems find out how difficult it will be to see an outside specialist. *You must not rely on a verbal communication. Instead, get something in writing prior to enrolling.*

A woman had a wonderful, caring internist. For financial reasons, she decided to change to an HMO thinking she could continue seeing her special physician. It was a rude awakening to discover her doctor was not on the HMO list of doctors. She found another physician after a long search, but her health declined steadily from then on.

Trying to save money by enrolling in an HMO could be the worst decision you ever make. The HMOs rarely refer to outside specialists, even though that type of specialist is not on their HMO list. The decision can be appealed but this necessitates a great amount of time and energy. Most patients don't feel up to doing this, which I'm sure the HMO administrators count on.

30. It is important to find out which hospital or hospitals you can use prior to enrolling in an HMO. You want to be sure the hospital is close and that you or a family member will not have to be taken a long distance for care. Be sure to ask if the plan will pay for the care in another hospital, if you have an emergency. They may not be willing to pay, but if the emergency is life threatening, you have a better case. Be sure to save any bills from another hospital or urgent care center. There have been some tragic cases where an HMO would not authorize care at a nearby hospital and insisted a patient go to one under contract with them. Some of the hospitals were at great distance resulting in much more serious problems and even deaths.

31. If you join an HMO and a specialist or procedure is not covered by the HMO or your insurance company and approval is denied, you can file a first-level appeal.

Most HMOs state in their rules how many days you have in which to file an appeal. It is often thirty to sixty days after you have received treatment or seen a specialist. You should save all the medical bills you have received, if you have had to go ahead with treatment that was not authorized. Also, you need to save a record of all the conversations you have had with HMO individuals and any correspondence you have had with them. It is a good idea to keep a telephone sheet to record dates, names of individuals contacted, and substance of conversations. If the first appeal is denied, try to find out the names of the people who denied it.

A ten-year-old boy was seen by a specialist in another state and after a two hour consultation and a muscle biopsy, a diagnosis was given to the parents. They had been told by their original doctors that their son had the lethal form of muscular dystrophy. You can imagine their relief when the specialist said it was a very mild form of a localized muscle disease. The parents had received prior authorization for the visit. However, after billing the insurance company, only ten percent of the bill was paid. The couple was appalled and said they would file a *first-level appeal*. They did not have a large income, but paid a sizeable monthly fee for their insurance coverage.

The first-level appeal was denied, so the feisty couple filed a *second-level appeal*. This meant considerable paper work and telephone calls. It also meant meeting with officers from the insurance company. The meeting turned out well and the specialist's bill was paid. The doctor greatly appreciated the couple's refusal to let the insurance company get by without adequate payment for the large amount of time she had spent with the boy.

32. **If the first-level appeal is denied, you can file a second-level appeal.** This too, will take considerable time and energy. However, the HMO and insurance companies should be forced to pay for the care you need.

33. **If you have paid for the HMO coverage through your employer or if your employer has paid all or part of it, you can file a complaint with the company's Human Resource department.** An employer should have more clout than you do as an individual. However, you may have to tread carefully at first and then later get more aggressive, if necessary. Some employers are great about standing up for their employees; others don't want to get into the health care battle.

34. **A certified letter to the medical director of an HMO about an excessive bill, with a request for a return**

receipt, may get results. A carbon copy sent to your senator or representative could help get a response from a member of the hospital staff.

A sixty-year-old woman dislocated her shoulder in a household accident. She went to the emergency room in the small town where she lived and the ER doctor ordered an X-ray. This confirmed the dislocation, and the man referred her to a local orthopedist. It took about six weeks for the hospital bill to arrive but when it did, it was outrageously padded. The woman was amazed and angry about the charges. After numerous calls and letters to the hospital administration and billing department, she sent copies of her letters to her state and federal representatives. Eventually, the billing department removed $1000 from her bill. The squeaky wheel does get the grease.

35. **As a last resort, if a bill, procedure, or specialist's care is denied, you may get action, if** *you state in a letter you will consult an attorney.* Some major lawsuits have been filed against HMOs when necessary care or procedures have been denied and unnecessary deaths occurred. As a result, the HMOs have been forced to pay large sums of money. Their administrators are extremely leery of lawyers and lawsuits.

One feisty mother wanted her seriously ill son to be seen by a specialist in another state. Not only did she hire an attorney to help her, but she also wrote letters of complaints to the newspapers. As a final resort, she enlisted the aid of friends to help picket the HMO office. She was ultimately allowed to have her son seen by the specialist and to be hospitalized for the needed tests.

36. Filing a complaint

Filing a complaint about poor medical care with your state HMO or insurance control board will help you and others. Each state has a division responsible for HMOs and insurance companies. In some states, the complaint should be made to the Department of Corporations. Complaint forms and instructions can also be obtained from a state's official Web site. Each state also has an HMO Hotline for complaints.

With some insurance plans, you can request an Independent Medical Review. This will take a lot of paperwork, but could be worthwhile and save you money. Some states also have special advocacy programs for individuals with insurance problems. There are some good advocacy groups that can be very helpful when you need advice and support.

Remember that you usually get what you pay for. Managed care is "assembly line" medicine. "Patients are 'processed' through hospitals, clinics, and doctors' offices as fast and as cheaply as possible."[1]

In California, the Health Insurance Counseling Program (HICAP) can be found by dialing toll-free 1-800-434-0222. An HMO Help Center is also available via the Internet at http://www.hmohelp.ca.gov or by dialing the toll-free number at 1-888-HMO-2219. Other states should have agencies such as these.

The phrase "Buyer Beware" is very applicable to HMOs and all health insurance companies.

---

[1] Head, Simon: *Bitter Harvest for Productive Labor Force*:-Los Angeles Times, 12/28/03, pg.M5.

37. Health Discount Cards

Some individuals are buying Health Discount Cards. These may not be of any value, so it is important to ask lots of questions about the specific benefits before purchasing one. There are many glitzy ads on TV, in the newspapers and mail by companies that want your business. I would be extremely careful about paying attention to any of these ads. (Only New Zealand and the U.S. allow drug companies to advertise.) Do lots of research before you spend your hard-earned money.

The new government health discount cards for low-income Medicare patients are not proving to be satisfactory, despite heavy advertising by the administration. This law was enacted December 8, 2003. The law is supposed to benefit Medicare beneficiaries whose income is not above 135 percent of the poverty line. This is $12,123 for single individuals and $16,362 for married individuals. (This was as of 2003 and will be adjusted.) Those at or below 100 percent of poverty will have to pay five percent co-insurance and above 100 percent will pay ten percent. As with many government programs, the program may be difficult to understand, so it should be carefully evaluated.

Caution is advised before signing up for any questionable drug discount program. Canadian drugs are being purchased by many individuals, but U.S. drug companies are battling to keep all Canadian drugs out of the U.S. They argue that there is no control over the quality of the drugs. Money rather than quality seems to be the drug companies' primary interest. *The profit margin of drug companies is the highest of any U.S. corporation.*

38. Referral to Specialists

It is important to know when your primary physician should refer you to a specialist. Many HMOs and insurance companies try to limit visits to specialists because of the added cost. An orthopedic surgeon should almost always treat problems such as bone and joint pain or an injury. A sprain may not be just a sprain and could require a cast or other treatment. Without the proper treatment, there could be prolonged pain or permanent injury. Back injuries should always be cared for by an orthopedic surgeon or a neurosurgeon, not a general doctor or physical therapist. If your primary doctor will not refer you to a specialist, see #31 about how to file a first-level appeal. You will probably have to push hard to get any action. There are multiple stories about the appeal process dragging out. Lawsuits have been filed and patients have died before being seen by a needed, outside specialist.

> An older woman slipped in her kitchen, hitting the refrigerator as she fell. She could hardly get up and was in great pain. When she called her primary doctor, the answering service said the doctor was out of town. The physician who was taking calls saw the woman and sent her to a physical therapist without ordering an X-ray. The smart physical therapist refused to give any treatment until X-rays of the chest and back were taken. It took some pushing and two or three days for this to be done. A cracked rib was seen on the X-ray. Physical therapy could have caused increased pain and disability and was not indicated.

****

A psychiatrist thought she had hurt her knee because of all the walking she did on a European trip. Her primary care doctor thought she had bursitis of the knee and treated her with injections into the joint. He did not refer her to an orthopedist, as he should have. No X-rays were taken and the doctor continued injecting her knee despite increasing pain and disability. The patient insisted on X-rays. The X-ray of the knee was negative, so an X-ray of the hip was taken. This showed marked degeneration of the bone and the woman was *finally* referred to an orthopedic surgeon. He recommended an immediate hip replacement. The surgery went well, as did the rehabilitation. The psychiatrist was angry that she had not insisted on seeing an orthopedist sooner. (Knee pain frequently comes from hip problems.)

CHAPTER SIX

Your Medical Records

The days of having a long-time family physician who knows you and your family are almost gone. In the past, your medical records were safe in your doctor's office; and if the doctor retired or died, another doctor usually took over. Now that medicine is so fragmented, it is important for each patient to keep copies of as many of his or her records as possible.

39. **Request and keep copies of all your medical records, test results, and reports or doctors' summaries in a file where you can find them.** Keeping these in order by date will help if a new physician needs to see them. If you have a special three-ring notebook for records, they can be easily found. Physicians retire, die, or sell their practices. Records may not be retained by the physician taking over the practice, so it is important that you keep copies of as many of your test results as possible. If you are to have surgery or are hospitalized for any reason, it is important to take along a summary of medical problems, surgeries, allergies, or reactions to anesthetics that you have had.

40. **Request that copies be made of any X-rays, CT scans and MRIs.** There will be a charge for this service and sometimes resistance from the hospital or office staff. However, it is your right to have these copies. Take them to doctors' appointments as needed. Most offices and hospitals keep these studies for seven years or less. It may be extremely important to have old X-rays or MRIs,

if a problem is detected. Without the old films, it would be difficult to know if the problem was previously present.

If you move to another city, it is extremely important to take X-rays and reports with you. It is often hard for a new doctor or hospital to obtain copies of old X -rays, CT scans, MRIs or reports. If you have had a serious health problem, such as a questionable mass in the breast or other area, baseline X-rays are extremely important to have and take with you to each follow-up appointment. That way, a comparison can be made between your old and new X-rays.

41. **Keep a summary of past medical problems with the dates and a list of any procedures you have had done.** Take this with you when you see a new doctor. If you have major medical problems, it is a good idea to keep a list in your purse or wallet. It is also important to always carry your physician's name and number, plus insurance or HMO information. If you are a grandparent and take a child to a doctor's appointment or the emergency room, you will need a copy of their parents' insurance and a note giving you permission to sign for treatment for the child.

There is now available a Medical Information Chip on which medical information can be stored: medications, allergy, immunization records, emergency phone numbers to contact, and even digital copies of X-rays and EKG results. The information can be updated as needed. The chip is available at: www.medinfochip.com and sells for seventy dollars.

CHAPTER SEVEN

Becoming Informed

Unless you are in the medical profession, it is often hard to separate fact from fiction. Even doctors may not be up-to-date about the latest medical facts. Asking lots of questions of different medical personnel is the best way to get information. There are some Internet sites, as from large clinics and medical schools, you should be able to trust. Unfortunately, even these do occasionally publish reports with errors. Newsletters from non-profit agencies for individuals with different medical problems offer some valuable information, but some may not be well documented. It is important to check if the information is written by an expert in that particular field of medicine.

42. **Reading medical journals can be risky for people without medical training**. There are erroneous reports, as in any published material. The Internet also has considerable incorrect information. It is important to read newspapers and magazines to learn facts, for example that some X-rays are being sent to India to be interpreted and there are medical transcriptions "farmed out" to typists in countries as far away as Pakistan! This happens more often than I would like to think and is troublesome. It is important to have your X-rays read by a physician your physician knows and trusts. *There can be grave errors in the interpretation of X-rays.*

   A college student was having problems with her menstrual periods and on graduation was referred to the head OB-Gyn doctor in a medical school in the city where she planned to move. The doctor in the medical school ordered X-rays of the young woman's head. The radiologist on reviewing the X-rays reported a tumor of the pineal gland. Surgery was advised.

Fortunately, a close relative was a physician connected with the medical school. She obtained the X-rays and had them reviewed by the head of the radiology department in another hospital. This radiologist was the author of a radiology text book and well-respected in his field. He looked carefully at the X-rays and said, "I don't see anything wrong with the patient's head." Later, the woman physician was talking to a pathologist friend, who worked in the medical school. The doctor was tired and complained she was having to look at many pineal glands that had been surgically removed. 'They were all normal," she said. "I wonder what is going on!"

43. **Always ask why a specific medicine, procedure, or lab test is needed**. There are basic tests that should be ordered when you have a physical examination. These include a complete blood count (CBC), urinalysis, tuberculin (TB) skin test and or a chest X-ray. More complex tests may need to be ordered dependent on any abnormal findings or complaints. *However, unless an adequate history is taken and a good physical examination done, lab tests should not be ordered.*

A thirty-five-year-old mother of three was feeling ill and saw her physician, a member of a large medical group. He took a short history and did a limited physical examination. Then he ordered an enormous numbers of tests, but said he didn't have a working diagnosis. When another physician was consulted, she couldn't understand why most of the tests had been ordered. They had little to do or nothing to do with the woman's complaints.

Batteries of tests are often ordered these days to save time for physicians and protect them from lawsuits. This is called "defensive medicine". Many physicians want to cover all possibilities, even totally unrealistic ones, so a patient won't have a reason to sue. In the long run, the old-fashioned practice of taking a complete history and doing a thorough physical examination saves time and money.

If a physician orders multiple tests, I would question why they are needed and what the physician is looking for. If a complete history and physical have not been done, I would insist that this be done prior to having many, perhaps unnecessary, tests. You may have to be assertive or change physicians, if your wishes are not respected.

44. **Ask about possible side effects for any drug prescribed**. Drugs may have side effects that are uncommon, but can cause problems. Some medications cause drowsiness; others may cause urinary retention (difficulty voiding), constipation, or a host of other symptoms. If you aren't comfortable with what the physician is saying, discuss the drug with a pharmacist you trust. Always check the label of a prescription you have filled to be sure it matches the doctor's prescription. It is important, too, to read the labels and check the contents of over-the-counter drugs. This is especially true for children or adults who take multiple medicines.

A woman was treated with the antibiotic, Augmentin, for an infection. Several weeks later she began to show signs of liver disease. Her doctor asked if she was taking any medication and when the answer was "No", he didn't ask about drugs she had taken recently. Repeated attempts were made to find the cause of her elevated liver tests with no success. Fortunately, the woman's husband, a professor of microbiology in a medical school, began to do some research. When he looked up the side-effects of Augumentin, the report said that elevated liver function tests occurred in a small number of cases. With this information, the woman's doctor stopped doing invasive tests. In time, the liver tests returned to normal and a liver biopsy was avoided.

45. **If you take multiple medications, if is important to check with a reliable pharmacist to be sure the drugs can all be taken together**. (Some university schools of pharmacy have numbers your physician can call to check on specific drugs.) Some medications can cause dangerous reactions when several or just one or two are taken together. If more than one doctor gives you a prescription, he or she may not be aware of other medications you are taking. They may not have asked or they may have asked but don't want to take the time to check if there could be dangerous interaction between drugs.

> One elderly woman was taking twenty-four medications, prescribed by different specialists. Her daughter discovered this and called the mother's primary doctor. He did not return her call, so she took all the bottles to her longtime, neighborhood pharmacist. He did research and found that several of the medications could interfere with each other and cause potential problems.

> The woman convinced her mother to find a different primary physician. It was his responsibility, she felt, to know what her mother was taking and check to see if the medicines could all be taken together.

It takes time to check multiple drugs and see if there are any interactions. Not all physicians are willing to take the time.

Elderly individuals who take several medications should write out a weekly chart listing: name, dose, and time of day the medicine should be taken. A dry-erase board or blackboard can be used. Pills can also be counted and put in containers that have a place for each day: Sat, Sun, Mon, Tues, Wed, Thurs, Fri. Family members or home health aides can do it, if seniors need help.

46. Always check to see if a medicine should be taken with food or on an empty stomach. Some medications, such as aspirin can cause irritation of the stomach lining and are best not to take on an empty stomach. A coated aspirin is available that is easier on the stomach.

Antibiotics should not be taken or prescribed for every cold or minor infection. They should be saved for infections that don't respond to bed rest, aspirin or Tylenol, and fluids. It is important to continue taking an antibiotic, when it has been prescribed, even though you feel better. An antibiotic should be prescribed for a specified period of time. Antibiotics should not be prescribed by a physician over the telephone. There is no possible way a physician can make a diagnosis by just talking to a patient.

Antibiotics should not be passed around among family or friends and expiration dates should always be checked. *Outdated tetracycline medications should not be taken but flushed down the toilet because they can cause liver damage.*

Some medications cause changes in blood counts or liver blood tests. If these medications are being taken, periodic blood counts or liver panels should be done. Some seizure medications and outdated antibiotics cause changes in liver tests. If these medications are taken, blood studies should be checked periodically to be sure the drugs did not or are not causing damage.

If drugs are purchased on-line, consumers should look for the seal that says "Verified Internet Pharmacy Practice Site". If you click on the seal, it will open a link to the National Association of Boards of Pharmacy. The Web site is http://www.nabp.net. The Food and Drug Administration (F.D.A.) has an 800 number, if you think a drug or pharmacy is not licensed. The number is 1-800-332-1088.

Prescription Assistance:

The Partnership for Prescription is a group composed of doctors, pharmaceutical companies, patient advocacy organizations, other healthcare providers and community groups. The purpose of the group is to help low-income patients obtain medicines, either at no cost or at a very low cost. Through their Web site 275 public and private patient assistance programs are available. The Web site is: www.pparx.org and the toll-free number is 1-888-477-2669.

Generic drugs:

Some individuals are leery of taking generic drugs and always want brand names. Advertising may play a part in this. Generic drugs are just the same as brand-name drugs and will save a patient considerable money. It has been noted that once a drug becomes generic it sometimes takes the drug company a while to up-date the labels, if there are any new warnings about side effects. However, you should discuss the side effects of any drugs you are taking with your physician or a pharmacist.

Performance-enhancing supplements:

Even though anabolic steroids and steroid precursors are illegal for athletes to use, protein powers and creatine are still being purchased at health food stores. These are not regulated by the Food and Drug Administration and may contain other substances: growth hormone, testosterone, or anabolic steroids. Also, the long-term effects are not known.

CHAPTER EIGHT

What is a Complete Physical Examination?

One of the most important diagnostic tools is becoming used less and less. More and more doctors are not doing complete histories and physicians prior to ordering large batteries of tests. (Medical students in many schools are not learning to take good histories or do complete physical examinations.) Most laboratory tests are unnecessary, if a complete work-up is done prior to tests being ordered. It takes time to obtain a detailed history and do a complete physical exanimation. Ordering lab work is much faster.

47. **For a physician to do a complete physical examination, a patient *must be* undressed down to shorts or underwear and wear a gown.** If this is not done, *important physical findings may be missed. No adequate examination can be done, if a patient is not undressed.* It is also hard to hear the heart and lungs through a gown, which is the practice of some physicians.

> I was examining children at a school and saw one little girl who was being followed for congenital heart disease by a well-known, local pediatrician. On looking at the child's back, I noted a moderately severe curvature of the spine (scoliosis). If this had not been detected and was allowed to progress, heart and lung damage could have resulted. "Why didn't Dr. R. find this", the mother asked? She answered her own question saying, "I guess it is because he never has me take off her blouse."

48. **A yearly urinalysis examination is important to look for infection, bleeding, signs of kidney disease, and diabetes**. *It may be necessary to check one more frequently, if a specific medical problem occurs.*

> A teenager was seen because she had a fever and felt ill. I couldn't find anything wrong after a thorough examination. A urine specimen and blood count were also normal. I asked the mother to bring the girl again the next day to be rechecked. Again there were no findings, so I requested another urine specimen.
>
> "But you just checked one yesterday", the mother said. "Yes", I said. "I won't charge you for looking at it, but I would like to look at another specimen." The girl returned from the bathroom with a specimen cup containing dark brown urine. Looking at it, I knew there was blood in the urine and the girl probably had glomerulonepritis. *(This is an extremely serious, but treatable kidney disease.)* The mother never complained about any other tests I wanted to do on her children and subsequently referred me many patients.

49. **Adults need yearly, routine blood tests: blood counts, cholesterol, fats and standard blood panels.** These panels include tests for blood sugar, liver studies, potassium, and similar things. Eye and hearing examinations should be done as needed. Beware of eye doctors (ophthalmologists), who have untrained aides do their refractions for glasses.

50. **A chest X-ray is advisable for adults every one to two years, particularly if the patient is a smoker.** Some health departments offer free chest X-rays and tuberculin skin tests. If a patient has been given BCG, as happens frequently in Asia, a tuberculin (TB) skin test will be positive and should not be given. Instead, a chest X-ray

each year would be important. (BCG is a weak dose of tuberculosis, so a patient can build up immunity or resistance to it). This is not recommended in the U.S.

Women should have a baseline mammogram at age forty or earlier, if there is a strong family history of breast cancer.

When there is a strong family history of cancer of the colon, a colonoscopy should be scheduled by age fifty or sooner, if a gastroenterologist recommends it. If there are problem with abdominal pain, diarrhea, or irritable bowel syndrome, your doctor may want this done before age fifty.

Pneumoccocal injections to guard against pneumonia are now advised for all individuals over age sixty-five or those with progressive disease that involve the lungs, such as Duchenne muscular dystrophy, and related disorders.

CHAPTER NINE

Medical Care for Children

Children are not little adults. Kids can become ill very quickly and all of their doctors should have pediatric training. If not serious consequences can occur.

51. **When you chose a pediatrician or family doctor, you want to be sure he or she relates to you, as well as your children.** You should also check to be sure the doctor is board-qualified or board-certified. Kids should be involved in their medical care, as much as possible when they are old enough to answer a doctor's questions or ask them. You also want to check and see what provisions are made to isolate sick children in the waiting room. Taking a new baby or healthy child for a check-up and sitting next to a child with a fever or one who is coughing or might be contagious is unwise.

It is important to find out at which hospital or hospitals the doctor has staff privileges and who will take care of your child, if an after hours emergency arises. Some doctors refer all parents to an emergency room after hours. Emergency room doctors have not had the same training as pediatricians or family doctors. They are usually o.k. for trauma or serious accidents, but for most children's medical problems their own pediatrician, family doctor, or an associate physician is needed.

Some doctors have more than one office, so you want to be sure the office near you is open when it is convenient for you, particularly if you work outside the house. Some doctors have evening and Saturday hours, so this is important to check.

Children and teens need a yearly, *complete* examination by a physician. Part of the examination should consist of questions about diet, sleep, medications taken, allergies, exercise, relationships with peers, school progress, and any worries or fears the youth may have. (Fluid intake, such as soft drinks, juice, and water are also important to be noted.) A doctor should talk to your child as much as possible if he or she is old enough to answer questions. If any doctor spends just five to ten minutes in the examining room and doesn't do a complete physical examination with a child undressed, it's time to find a new physician. A complete examination should include inspecting the body all over, not just above the waist.

52. **Try not to take more than one small child at a time to an appointment.** Your doctor will thank you and do a better job with the child he or she is examining. An older child can take a book and sit quietly in the waiting room. Each child needs his or her own time to be examined. Other children in the examining room are potential distractions or noise makers. Loud laughter or noise in the waiting room may not be enjoyed by the staff or others waiting. Waiting room manners are as important to teach as table manners.

53. **Carry a copy of your children's immunizations with you at all times.** This is particularly important, if you are traveling and an accident or injury occurs. Check yearly to be sure the immunizations are up-to-date. Not all doctors are careful about looking at the immunization record when they do a yearly physical examination. *Grandparents, who have part or full-time care of grandchildren, should also carry a copy of their grandchildren's immunizations.*

Parents of children with autism are often reluctant to have any younger children immunized. They fear that the autism of their older child was caused by the multiple immunizations now being given. Several comprehensive studies have been done which report that there is *no* connection between autism and immunizations.

54. Insist a child be seen by a physician before antibiotics are prescribed. When antibiotics are prescribed over the telephone, without a child being seen, a serious infection could be missed. Meningitis can develop very quickly, so a child or teenager should always be seen when there is cause for concern or a high, unexplained fever.

> A two-year old developed a croupy cough and two different prescriptions for antibiotics were called in to a pharmacy by the child's doctor. He did not see the child. The little boy didn't improve after two or three weeks, so the parents made an appointment with the pediatrician. Another doctor was taking his place that day and after examining the child, she ordered a chest X-ray. To everyone's amazement, the X-ray showed a safety pin in the child's windpipe (trachea). The parents remarked that the little boy was always putting things in his mouth and must have found a safety pin on the floor. Somehow, the safety pin ended up in his windpipe. An ear, nose, and throat doctor saw the child that day and removed the pin in the operating room. The croupy cough disappeared.

55. Post the number of the local poison center or the national one, 1-800-222-1222 and the number of your child's doctor by your telephone. Be sure babysitters know where to find the numbers. Also, post the number and location of the closest hospital. Your babysitter needs to know what to do in a medical emergency and be able to communicate with emergency personnel. The babysitter should know where you keep medical supplies and when to call the child's doctor.

Every babysitter or caretaker should know what to do if a child is choking or stops breathing. CPR courses are available at hospitals and the Red Cross. There is also a good CPR video available at www.CPR.com.

A couple went on a ski trip and left their two children with a non-English speaking babysitter. Fortunately, a neighbor agreed to check on the children. The third day after the parents left for vacation, the kind woman stopped by and discovered that the two-year-old boy was quite ill. The babysitter had not called the pediatrician. It was a Saturday afternoon, so the doctor's office was closed. However, the doctor immediately answered the call and was at the child's bedside within thirty minutes. She found a very ill little boy and immediately took him to the hospital. The parents were unable to be contacted because they had moved hotels and not left their new number. The child had severe pneumonia by chest X-ray and had to be kept in the hospital several days. The parents were not found even after many telephone calls. When they returned from their vacation, their son was recovering from the pneumonia, eating well, and playing. The doctor had taken him home, as soon as he was well enough to be there. The parents were apologetic and said they would be more careful the next time they went on vacation!

56. **Insist that your child have a yearly urinalysis to look for infection, bleeding, or diabetes. Even babies and small children need a yearly examination of the urine.** If there is a family history of kidney or urinary problems, extra attention should be paid. *An unexplained fever in a child always merits an examination of the urine.*

A three-month-old child had a high fever. The doctor couldn't find a cause but checked a urine specimen. Pus cells and other signs of infection were seen and a pediatric urologist was called. The baby was found to have abnormalities of both tubes (ureters) from the kidneys to the bladder. Subsequently, two surgeries were performed to control the problem. The first doctor may have saved the baby's life.

57. Insist that your child have a tuberculin (TB) skin test every one to two years. This is particularly important in states where there is an increased incidence of tuberculosis. California has a particularly high incidence. Treatment is available for tuberculosis, but if it is not detected, it can spread throughout the body and cause what is termed, "miliary TB". Death can result.

A three-year-old was admitted to a children's hospital because of on-going weight loss, poor appetite, and cough. For some reason, a chest X-ray and TB skin test were not done. The attending staff thought the child had a heart problem because they had heard a heart murmur. Several days after the child was admitted to the hospital, she died suddenly. An autopsy was done which revealed miliary tuberculosis. The doctors-in-charge were embarrassed and also concerned that everyone who had been near the boy had been exposed to tuberculosis.

58. Insist that an eye chart be read each year in the primary doctor's office. If a child squints, is cross eyed, "wall eyed", or holds books close to the face, an eye examination by a pediatric ophthalmologist is needed. If a child wants to sit very close to the TV, he or she could need glasses. Also if a child has frequent headaches, the eyes should be examined. It could be that too much time is spent watching TV or using a computer.

59. Insist that hearing be checked yearly in your primary doctor's office.

A little girl had not started speaking, and her pediatrician decided she should be seen by a speech therapist. He called a physician, who specialized in treating children with disabilities, to ask the name of a good one. When the specialist asked if the child's hearing had been checked, the pediatrician said, "Oh that's a good idea." Subsequently, the little girl was found to be partially deaf.

Children can develop severe ear infections without a fever. If a child is not eating and is crying a lot or pulling at one or both ears, suspect an ear infection and see a physician. Sometimes kids will tilt their head to the side where an ear is painful and infected.

A two-year-old and his mother spent the night with the grandmother. The little boy cried and was restless all night. His mother thought it was teething but the grandmother was sure the little boy had an ear infection. Early the next morning, they saw the child's doctor. He confirmed that the eardrum was about to burst.

****

A little girl with cerebral palsy had a prolonged seizure (convulsion) and was taken to a large medical school hospital. The seizures were finally brought under control, but no cause was found. The discharge diagnosis was "constipation". The day after the discharge, the mother took her daughter to see the specialist who followed the child for the cerebral palsy. After a thorough examination, the doctor asked the mother what the hospital doctors had said about the little girl's ears. "She has bad ear infections on both sides that look as if they have been there for several days", the physician said. "Oh", said the excellent mother, "I stayed with her the whole time she was in the hospital and of the eight doctors who saw her, no one did a complete physical or checked her ears!"

60. Nurse practitioners do a fine job of giving general pediatric information and working with doctors, but by law a physician must see a child at an office visit. Some big stores are starting to open "retail-based clinics" staffed by nurses. This is worrisome.

A mother with a child who had weak muscles was pleased that a specific diagnosis had been made by a specialist on her five-year-old son. She was concerned, however, that the child fatigued so easily. She told the specialist that she thought her pediatrician was good and yet on questioning, the mother said no basic tests had been done since the boy was two-years-old. Most of the care had been given by a nurse practitioner. The mother thought the child was allergic because he wheezed a lot and had eczema, but no allergy tests had been done; nor had the child been seen by a pediatric allergist. Tests for thyroid function, diabetes, anemia, and infection had not been done. The specialist made a list of things she would recommend and the mother promised to find another physician who saw the children and did not leave the care to others. Unfortunately, when a patient has one disorder, such as muscle weakness, every other symptom is assumed to be part of that disorder.

61. A child or teenager should wear a Medic Alert bracelet, if he or she has a serious allergy or chronic medical condition. The Medic Alert number is 1-800-

432-5378 and their web site is: http://www.medicalert.org. The staff keeps an up-to-date file on each individual registered with them and they are on-call twenty-four-hours a day, seven days a week. Immediate emergency information can be provided when a physician calls.

If a child has a serious allergic problem, epinephrine or an "Epi-Pen" should always be on hand. Parents and caretakers must know how and when to use it. School nurses should also be trained and teachers must be aware of the allergy.

> One mother was taught how to use epinephrine because her child was highly allergic to bees. The little boy was stung by a bee, but, rather than use the epinephrine as she had been taught, the mother carried it with her when she rushed the child to the doctor's office. Valuable time was lost, which could have resulted in the child's death. Fortunately, the doctor saw the child right away and epinephrine was given, along with other treatment.

62. Grandparents or relatives who have part or full-time care of children or who might take a child to see a doctor may need to carry a letter stating they are allowed to do this. Some doctors will not see a child, except for a true emergency, unless the adult bringing in the child for care provides a signed statement or proxy from the custodial parent. If the parents are divorced, problems can sometimes arise if the non-custodial parent takes a child to the doctor. A medical consent-to-treat form can be obtained at www.acep.org. This form gives a caregiver the ability to authorize treatment in an emergency situation.

Grandparents who have part or full-time care of their grandchildren should keep up-to-date medical records. They need to always carry a copy of their grandchildren's immunizations and lists of any allergies or special medical problems. If there is a family history of genetic or medical problems, a grandparent can play an important part in helping a physician or medical team make a correct diagnosis.

> One grandmother had a particular interest in family history and put together a beautiful scrapbook with family pictures and medical histories covering several generations. Because of her research, a physician was able to make a diagnosis on a grandchild that had not even been considered. A new treatment was available, which would not have been offered without the grandmother's research.

63. It is important for parents to know when they have to become *assertive* with their child's doctor. Most parents don't want to have to challenge a doctor, but sometimes there is no other choice when a child's health, or even life is at stake.

> A seven-year-old boy had a fever of 102 degrees and seemed quite ill. His mother called the pediatrician's office and asked for an appointment. The doctor's nurse said, "Dr. R. doesn't see a child unless they have a temperature of 102 degrees for four days!"

> The boy continued to have a fever that went up and down. He also had a cough and wasn't eating well. The mother didn't want to seem pushy, but her husband was out of town and she was becoming more and more concerned. At the urging of a doctor who was visiting a nearby friend, the mother insisted on an appointment with the doctor. He examined the boy but said he couldn't find any reason to worry. No lab work or chest X-ray were done and the fever continued intermittently for nine days. The visiting

doctor again urged the mother to insist that a chest X-ray be taken. If that was negative, she said a blood count and urinalysis should be done. Other tests would be needed, if these were all negative.

No child should be allowed to have an intermittent fever for several days without a thorough work-up being done to find the cause of the fever. Pneumonia, meningitis, and other serious diseases can be missed.

Diagnostic Tips for Children

- Before an eye doctor is allowed to probe an obstructed tear duct in an infant, it is worthwhile to try gentle massage at the inner corner of the eye and warm compresses. Often this will open up the tear duct and make surgery unnecessary.

- Boy babies who are not circumcised often develop large collections of a cheesy secretion called smegma under the foreskin. The foreskin should be gently pulled back and the smegma removed. (One intensive care doctor thought a collection of smegma was a tumor and was appalled when I removed the "tumor"!)

- Little children stick foreign bodies in every orifice: the nose, ears, mouth, vagina, and rectum. If pus is coming out of a child's orifice, think of a foreign body.

- Constipation in children can mimic the pain of an appendicitis. Two-year- olds who prefer milk to food are particularly at risk for constipation. Apples and bananas are constipating. Children with muscle weakness are particularly prone to constipation.

- A colicky baby may be allergic to milk. Breast-fed babies may be allergic to milk products the mother has ingested.

- An asthmatic child may be allergic to milk or other foods: eggs, chocolate, citrus, fish, nuts, or wheat.

- A child who has a fever that comes and goes for several days should always be checked by a pediatrician or family doctor. In addition, a urinalysis, blood count, and chest X-ray are indicated. Pneumonia can be difficult to diagnose because there are times when it is present and yet nothing abnormal can be heard in a child's chest.

- Girls should have a urological work-up after two urinary infections. Boys should have a urological work-up after the first urinary tract infection.

- Bed wetters should be seen by a pediatric urologist after age seven.

Preparing a Child for a Visit to the Emergency Room

1. Be sure your pediatrician or family doctor knows you are on you way to an E.R with your child.

2. Talk to your child, if he or she is alert, and try to explain what will happen.

3. Insist that a physician see your child.

4. Try to be patient and cooperative, but there are times when you have to make your presence known, particularly if it is a real emergency.

5. If your child needs to go to the bathroom, check to see if a urine specimen is needed.

6. If a lumbar puncture is to be done or stitches are needed, some children act more mature, if their

parents are not in the room. Also, the doctor may be more relaxed.

7. Carry a copy of your child's immunizations record with you, in case a tetanus shot is needed.

8. If a child has ingested a poisonous substance, drug, or poisonous plant, take along the box, pill bottle, or plant.

CHAPTER TEN

Special Needs Care

Multiple resources are available for individuals with special needs or disabilities. Many of these are difficult to locate or difficult to access because of layers of bureaucracy. Patients with disabilities often have to be quite vocal to have their medical needs met. However, there are some good advocacy programs.

64. Special Needs Clinics

Each state has free clinics for children with special needs. The care received is quite variable. The advantage of clinics is:

A. **You can meet other parents whose children have special needs.**

B. **Several medical professionals should be available for consultation.**

The major disadvantage of clinics is that a comprehensive history and physical examination can not be done in a clinic setting. Also a relationship with a single physician can not be established. In most state clinics, a child is seen for just a short time and not undressed, so it is important that another physician be seen regularly for a thorough examination. Physical therapy and occupational therapy can be received in school programs, even if parents prefer not to attend the free clinics. Some physical and occupational therapists don't let parents know this because they like the children to be seen in the clinics.

Individuals need a primary doctor who looks not only at their disability but at general health needs. Routine health care; urinalysis, blood counts, vision, hearing, and immunizations may be overlooked, if adequate time is not spent by a physician with a patient. Many patients with disabilities complain that every problem they have is immediately thought to be due to their disability, when it may be caused by something entirely different.

65. **Medical schools have special clinics for many disorders**. These have an attending staff doctor who consults briefly after a patient has been examined by a medical student or young doctor-in-training. If you want to see the staff doctor, an appointment should be made directly with his or her secretary. If a medical student or resident starts to do the examination in the private doctor's office, you should make it very clear that you have an appointment with the staff doctor, not a doctor-in-training.

66. **Special medical equipment needs are covered by some insurance plans, if a physician's prescription for the equipment is obtained.** The Muscular Dystrophy Association will buy some equipment for patients with neuromuscular conditions, so a call should be made to the local MDA office to see what help is available. The Muscular Dystrophy Family Foundation is very good about trying to help with equipment needs for patients who have a disorder falling under their umbrella. There are about twenty different disorders that are in their list of conditions to be aided. Their number is 1-800-544-1213 and their Web site is www.mdff.org. Some state programs pay for needed equipment, if you have a prescription from a physician. Considerable time, energy,

and paperwork will usually be needed before any equipment is obtained. Used equipment can often be purchased either through newspaper ads or through different agencies. Used vans can be purchased through van companies or agency newsletters. The Disabled Dealer at 1-800-588-5099 publishes a monthly newsletter of used vans and other equipment for sale. Their Web site can be viewed at: www.disableddealer.com.

A Web site that offers information and resources for children with disabilities can be found at http://www.kidstogether.org. Medical expense relief for kids with disabilities is offered at a Web site: http://www.firsthandfoundation.org.

67. High Risk insurance can be obtained for individuals with a disability or major health problem. The National Underwriters Company publishes a yearly list of all the insurance companies that write high-risk insurance. This list is available for about $9.95 by calling 1-800-543-0874. With this insurance you will have high deductibles and large premiums, but at least you will have insurance, which everyone needs in these days of high medical and hospital costs.

Another way to get insurance, if you are high risk, is under a state's health insurance "Risk Pool". Thirty states have these risk pools. A good summary is found at the Web site: http://www.healthinsurance.org/riskpoolinfo.html or in the Appendix.

If you are changing jobs or have lost a job, it is important to keep any insurance coverage that you have had. This is particularly true if you have a disability or major health problem. The COBRA law was passed in 1985 and "requires most employers with group health plans to offer employees the opportunity to continue temporarily their group health care coverage under their employer's plan if their coverage otherwise would cease due to termination, layoff, or other change in employment status". The Web site at http://www.cobrainsurance.net gives a good summary of COBRA insurance.

Beware of Insurance Scams

There are many individuals and companies that sell fraudulent insurance.

Warnings are issued about the following:

- A health insurance policy costing twenty-five percent or less than the standard, gives generous benefits, and also has a large provider network.

- Insurance companies that have names similar to reputable ones.

- Companies that will cover individuals with serious illnesses.

- A company saying it is not licensed in your state and that this is not necessary.

- Companies that do not require a preadmission physical examination.

If you have any doubt about an insurance company, call your state board of insurance. (See appendix). There is also a good Web site you can check: www.insurancefraud.org

CHAPTER ELEVEN

Emergency Medical Care

Emergency rooms are becoming increasingly crowded because some doctors are refusing to see welfare patients or they are not taking new patients. ER doctors should be seeing true emergencies, not patients with the flu, colds, coughs, or diaper rashes. If you have an emergency, you want the ER team to see you or a loved one immediately. In addition, emergency room care is extremely expensive, if the cost is not covered by welfare or insurance.

68. Emergency room doctors should never be used for general medical care, particularly for children.

Part of making a correct diagnosis is having some in-depth knowledge about a patient. If an emergency room is used for colds, coughs, or problems that should be seen in a doctor's office, the cost will be much more and the care may be fragmented or given by an overworked, tired emergency room physician. Also a great many unnecessary tests may be ordered because the doctor does not know the patient.

> A twenty-year-old, Alexis, was traveling several hundreds of miles to her parents for Christmas when she developed severe pain in her chest. She was stressed, felt very anxious, had a bad cough and cold, and at work had been sitting for many hours at a computer. She stopped at a hospital emergency room that was listed on her health plan brochure because she was becoming more and more anxious. There she was seen by a triage nurse who ordered a large battery

of tests. Six hours later, Alexis still had not been seen by a physician. By 2:00 A.M., she was so exhausted and felt so ill that she left the emergency room and drove to her parents' home. *Calls were never received from the hospital regarding her test results.* The results were obtained a week later when her former pediatrician called the hospital and obtained the results. They were all negative. The bill was enormous but was finally reduced because of multiple letters to the hospital CEO by the patient, her parents, and the pediatrician. No apology was received from any administrator for the multiple, unnecessary tests ordered by the nurse without a doctor's examination.

The diagnosis her former pediatrician made on taking a telephone history was that Alexis had a severe cold and cough, and her chest pain was due to stress and sitting at the computer for long hours. The six hours spent in the E.R., the multiple tests, and big bill could have been avoided had a physician seen her initially, taken an adequate history, and done even a quick physical.

69. When a patient is seen in an emergency room, it is important that the E.R. staff and doctor are given:

- Insurance information

- Treating doctors and their telephone numbers

- Family members to contact, if needed, and their telephone numbers

- A list of medicines you are taking or the actual bottles of medicine

- A list of any surgeries or medical procedures you have had

- Information about allergies and any drug reactions

70. **If a patient has a stroke or life-threatening disorder, an E.R. doctor needs to know if lifesaving measures are wanted or if an individual does not want to be resuscitated or put on life support.** The initials, DNR, are important to know. They mean "Do Not Resuscitate". A small card or typewritten note should be carried in a wallet or purse and a relative or friend should be aware of your wishes. Also everyone should have a Living Will or hand-written instructions that no lifesaving measures such as life support machines, I.V.s, or tube feedings are wanted.

71. **Ambulance drivers and paramedics also need to know a patient's wishes.** Some individuals keep a "Vial of Life" posted by their phone or on their refrigerator. This gives instructions about whether or not they want to be resuscitated following a major stroke, coma, or a life-threatening accident. The Vial of Life form and logo can be downloaded from the Internet at http://www.mypreciouskid.com/vial2.html.

CHAPTER TWELVE

Urgent Care and Surgical Outpatient Centers

Urgent care facilities have sprung up in many areas and any licensed physician can open one. They are not as carefully regulated by state agencies, as are hospital emergency rooms, so the care may range from excellent to poor. Also, cost may be considerably more than seeing a doctor in his or her private office.

72. **Knowing a patient's medical history is extremely important**. If a patient is seen for just a quick visit, a detailed history and complete examination can not be done. If a patient is from out-of-town, a follow-up examination may not be possible.

> A family was traveling when their teenage son became ill. They stopped at an urgent care center where a physician did a quick examination. Blood work was ordered and on receiving the results, the doctor said the youth had diabetes. He prescribed some medicine, which fortunately the parents did not let their son take. The medicine could have caused a severe reaction. Instead, the parents drove all night and saw the boy's pediatrician the next morning. She found a large patch of pneumonia in the teenager's lungs and prescribed antibiotics and bed rest. Further tests showed no evidence of diabetes.

73. **Urgent care centers, or as some call them, "the doc in the box", may be okay for a nosebleed, sprain, cut, or**

minor injury. However, a private doctor's office or the emergency room of a well-established, reputable hospital would be preferable. *Eye injuries should ALWAYS be seen by an eye doctor (ophthalmologist) or at a specialty eye hospital.*

> A college student came home for Christmas vacation with a bad cold and cough so her mother took her to a nearby urgent care center. The doctor spent about ten minutes with the girl and prescribed an antibiotic. The mother asked the doctor, as they were leaving; if her daughter's ears were o.k. (The girl had a past history of many ear infections.) "Oh," said the doctor, "I didn't look at them. Let me see!"

74. The Association of Ambulatory Healthcare regulates and/or monitors some urgent care centers. If you have a complaint about care you have received, you may contact the Joint Commission on Accreditation of Health Care Organizations (JCAHO) either by phone at their general telephone number which is not toll-free: 1-630-792-5000 or via their Web site at: http://www.jcaho.org. There are no strict state or federal standards for urgent care centers, as there are for hospital emergency rooms.

Ambulatory or Surgical Outpatient Centers

More and more surgical procedures are being done in outpatient centers. The good thing about this is that hospital infections should not be a problem. However, the down side is that not all the centers are clean or well equipped, and the anesthesia may be given by a nurse anesthetist or an M.D. who does not have his or her boards in anesthesia. This is extremely worrisome and some tragic deaths have occurred. If you are advised to have surgery in one of these centers, I would check the center out very carefully. You particularly want to find out the qualifications of the individual who will give the anesthesia. The American Association of Ambulatory Surgery Centers, at www.aaawsc.org, states that their centers are licensed and monitored by federal and state agencies. However, there is concern that some of the procedures performed in these centers should be done in hospitals where teams of professionals are available. There are 4,600 centers in the U.S., and large corporate hospital chains are buying many of these.

CHAPTER THIRTEEN

Hospital Care

Most people have a fear of being hospitalized because horror stories abound about poor care. With the present fragmentation of medicine, it is important for patients to know how to find good hospitals and insist on the best care. Knowing a few basic principals can make the difference between receiving good and mediocre, or life-threatening care.

75. **Big teaching hospitals are fine for unusual, complicated problems, if a conscientious, caring staff physician is in charge of your case.** If not, your care may be fragmented and left to inadequately trained medical students, interns, or residents, who are young doctors-in-training.

> One older woman did a great deal of research to find the best orthopedic surgeon for a needed hip replacement. The surgery went well, but the orthopedist visited her only twice after the surgery. He had several partners and one did see her occasionally. The rest of the woman's care was left to whatever doctor-in-training was on call that day. Fortunately, no problems developed. If there had been problems or complications, they could easily have been overlooked by the residents, who were not training to be orthopedic surgeons. Not only was her care inadequate, but *private, attending doctors are required by law to see their hospital patients at least every twenty-four-hours and write a daily note in the*

chart. Following major surgery, care must be provided by the operating surgeon or one of his or her partners.

NOTE: Because many laboratory tests are ordered these days during most hospital admissions, it is very important that a patient find out the results before discharge. When tests have to be sent to an outside laboratory or a special testing center, the results may take some time to come back. Often a patient is discharged before the results are received. If there is no follow-up by the patient's physician, a diagnosis or important result may be overlooked.

A child was seen as a follow-up to an out-of-state university hospital workup for muscle weakness. Multiple tests were preformed, but no diagnosis given. The parents were very discouraged and asked if I would obtain the records and review them. The child's medical records were voluminous and took many hours to review. However, the diagnosis seemed clear once the laboratory tests were reviewed. The results had apparently been received after the boy was discharged. I called the chief of the pediatric neuromuscular service at the out-of-state hospital and went over the findings with him. He agreed with my diagnosis and was much embarrassed that there had been no follow-up. The parents were very grateful I had found a diagnosis, because there was treatment for this rare neuromuscular disease.

76. **With the current nursing shortage, it is wise, if financially possible, to hire your own private duty nurse following a major surgery.** Otherwise, your care may be left to untrained aides and serious problems overlooked. Your primary physician or the operating surgeon may be able to give you the names of good private duty nurses. You can call the hospital nursing

office for referrals or look in the Yellow Pages under "Nursing Services". Friends may also have suggestions.

If it is not financially possible to hire a private duty nurse, plan to have a family member or friend stay with you at all times. If there is a problem, the hospital staff can be alerted.

77. **If a hospital admission is planned, a patient should have a signed and notarized "Living Will" or "Advanced Health Care Directive."** These forms can be downloaded from the Internet at: http://www.ilrg.com/forms/states/medicaldirective.html. (Each state has its own specifications, so it is necessary to specify your particular state). There is also a Web site at: www.agingwithdignity.org or you can call: 1-888-594-7437. The documents give instructions to health care providers about your wishes regarding what you want done in the event of a stroke, coma, or life-threatening disorder. If you have a horror of being kept alive by machines after a serious accident or illness, your wishes must be recorded on this form. Some local medical societies will send you a Living Will form. There is usually a minimal charge. These can be filled in, signed, and notarized. Your primary doctor and a close relative should have copies and everyone should have a signed copy in a safe deposit box. Advanced Health Care Directives can also be found at: www.mckweb.com/Advanced%2Directive.html. The Web site: www.medicaldirective.org can be accessed for documents giving directions about what you want as to: feeding tubes, respirators, resuscitation, and kidney dialysis.

78. **Prior to any surgery, treatment for cancer or serious medical problem, a second opinion should be sought.** If you are seeing a specialist who is considered one of the best in a field, you might ignore this advice. Even then

you might feel more comfortable about having a second opinion. However, "doctor shopping" can create problems because there are often different approaches and treatments for specific conditions.

If you have had a tumor removed or a muscle biopsy, it is important that a second opinion be sought regarding the diagnosis. There are many errors in the reading of pathology slides. Good general pathologists admit that they don't get training in all areas. Slides can be sent to specialists who have training in special areas: cancer, muscle disorders, or diseases of the skin and bones. There may or may not be a charge for this review, but it could make the difference in the diagnosis. Your life and future health care could be changed by insisting that a review be done.

> A woman had surgery for abdominal pain because it was believed she had ovarian cancer. The hospital where the surgery was done was one that had a reputation for giving average, but not outstanding care. The patient was told there was some question whether the ovary was cancerous or just cystic. She accepted this and decided to try alternative medicine, rather than chemotherapy. When she told this to a physician friend at a women's meeting, the physician said, "Have you had the pathology slides reviewed by a pathologist in an outstanding medical center?" No", the patient said, "I didn't know you could do that". The physician made some phone calls and gave the woman the name and telephone number of the head of the department in a major, eastern medical school. He had an outstanding reputation and was the physician who cared for a friend, who was a doctor's wife.

There are many different courses of treatment these days for the same problems, so your options should be carefully researched. An example is the current treatment for breast cancer. Some specialists advocate local incision of the tumor with no other treatment. Others advocate X-ray, chemotherapy, mastectomy, or a combination of the three. This can be very confusing, so a great deal of networking or research by reliable professionals is needed to receive the best treatment. *It could make the difference in your life.*

79. Follow instructions carefully for tests or procedures. If your doctor says not to eat anything after midnight prior to surgery, a procedure, or test, heed his or her advice. If you have eaten immediately prior to receiving an anesthetic, it could be life-threatening. Also, if you stuff yourself with food just before midnight you could be in big trouble. Food in the stomach can be vomited up into the lungs, if you are given an anesthetic, and cause great problems or even death. Some laboratory tests should be done when you have not eaten past midnight. Otherwise, the results will not be accurate.

80. If you are to have a surgical procedure, such as a breast biopsy or mastectomy, it is wise to write "Wrong side" with a felt-tip pen on the side where the operation is not to be performed. Surgeons do occasionally operate on the wrong side. There have been some tragic cases, where for example, a diseased kidney was to be removed and instead the good kidney was taken out.

81. If you are in the hospital for a major problem, there may be a time when you or a relative will have to become very assertive to stay in either the intensive care unit or the regular hospital. There are different levels of care in hospitals and if you have been seriously ill or had a major operation, you do not want to be moved to a floor where the care is given mostly by aides. These are called step-down units.

A thirty-eight-year old man cut his right big toe badly while he was on vacation. After returning home, he noticed that his right knee was swollen. He thought he had just twisted it and didn't start to worry until it became red and painful. Then he went to the local hospital emergency room and after a long wait was seen by a physician. The doctor gave him some medicine for the pain and sent him home. When the man started running a fever, his wife insisted they go back to the emergency room. By this time, he was so ill that he was admitted to the hospital. It took several days for an orthopedic surgeon to be called by the general medical doctor who was treating him. An MRI of the knee was taken and showed a layer of pus above the kneecap. For some reason, the orthopedist waited a few days before he drained the knee in the operating room. Instead, he kept the patient on intravenous fluids and antibiotics; even though the man was running a high fever and draining the knee would have released the pus. Two days after the knee was drained in the operating room, when the man was better but still ill, a clerk came into the room and said, "We're moving you today to the step-down unit." The man's feisty wife, a doctor's daughter, was there and she said, "No, you are not!" It took more strong words from the wife to keep her husband from being moved. She said, "I am prepared to go to the head administrator of the hospital, if necessary." Fortunately, the wife's words kept her husband from being moved until he was much better.

If you are hospitalized and told you are being discharged before you feel well enough to go home, you or a family member may have to get very assertive. If you are discharged too early, you may quickly get into trouble and have to return to the hospital. These days, the HMOs and insurance companies want you out of the hospital as soon as possible to save money. *Their goal is not good patient care, but increasing their own net worth.*

Skilled Nursing Facilities (SKF)

Skilled nursing facilities are available in many hospitals. They vary from good to bad. Patients who do not need intensive nursing by RNs are transferred to these units. Since the care can be poor, a family member or friend should be available to help with any needs. The food is often not too palatable, so food from outside could be welcome, depending on the medical condition.

CHAPTER FOURTEEN

College Health Care

When kids go away to college, most parents breathe a sigh of relief that they no longer have to be completely in charge. Many worry though about what will happen with their kid's new-found freedom. For some young people, this freedom means drinking too much, sleeping too little, and eating a poor diet. If this happens, resistance can be lowered and illness will take its toll. So, the college health service is as important to research, as the college or university.

82. **It is very important that young people have their immunizations brought up to date before they leave for college.** Most colleges now require a meningococcal vaccine prior to admission. In addition, several states: California, Connecticut, Delaware, Florida, Georgia, Indiana, Maryland, Missouri, New York, North Carolina, Oklahoma, Pennsylvania, Tennessee, Virginia, and Wisconsin have laws mandating that college students receive the vaccination, unless a release is signed.

If a college student has any kind of special medical problems, the student's doctor should send a letter to the college health service. Also, a letter should be given to the student to keep and show to doctors, as needed.

Colleges and universities vary in the health services they offer their students. A few smaller colleges have no health services. Before going off to college, both students and parents should find out exactly what is provided in the way of health care at the college and what the costs will be for routine care and emergency care. No two colleges offer the same benefits. Many college health services offer general health care for colds, minor injuries, and birth control; however, the majority don't offer medical care for serious medical or surgical problems and/or major accidents. Students are referred to private doctors or hospital emergency rooms.

83. **Many college students will still be covered by their parents' health insurance policies.** It is wise to check and be sure this is true, particularly if the college or university is out of state. This should be done prior to a student leaving for college. If the student is not full-time or is overage, a policy may not provide coverage. These days, health insurance is a very important part of getting good medical care.

84. **Health insurance for college students can be obtained through some of the colleges or through insurance companies, such as Aetna.** A few colleges require the students to buy the school's health plans. A health care consultant, Stephen Beckley, has a Web site that compares health care coverage for college and university students. It is www.slba.com

Before a student graduates from college, it is wise to check their health insurance to sure they will be covered until they find a job or decide to go on for more education. A policy to cover this time is called a "Bridge Policy". There is an insurance called GradMed at www.gradmed.com that covers college graduates. The insurance is under the American Insurance Administrators. This insurance will not cover any conditions that were pre-existing, even though the previous policy may have covered it. This policy is not renewable if a job opportunity doesn't work out. COBRA insurance is another option. However, a graduating student may be able to get a less expensive individual policy through a big company such as Blue Cross or Blue Shield.

85. If you are not sure about the quality of the college student health service, it is a good idea to do some research and get the name of a good general doctor or internist near the college. If there is an emergency, it could be better to use this physician rather than relying on the student health service. If the reputation of the health service is poor, I would urge all parents of college students to be sure their kids seek private medical care in a community near the college.

One college freshman at a major university was seen in the student health service because she was felt very ill. Tonsillitis was diagnosed and the girl was sent back to her dorm with some penicillin. It was a Friday afternoon and her roommate had left for the weekend. The girl became quite anxious because she felt extremely ill and was having great difficulty swallowing. Fortunately, the girl's former pediatrician had relocated near the university. After receiving an urgent call from the student's parents, the doctor quickly sped to the dorm and found her former patient to be extremely ill. She put in an emergency call to the doctor-on-call at the student health service and insisted that the student be hospitalized. The pediatrician's diagnosis was infectious mononucleosis, not tonsillitis. Lab tests confirmed her diagnosis. The greatly enlarged tonsils that occur with some cases of mononucleosis can cause airway obstruction, which can be very dangerous.

CHAPTER FIFTEEN

Senior Medical Care

As individuals are living longer and longer in the U.S., it has become increasingly important to know how and where to obtain the best senior health care and how to pay for it. Medicare has been an important program for seniors and in general is well run, although the amounts paid to many doctors are not adequate.

86. **Medical care has become so expensive that it is important to know how and when to apply for Medicare.** Applying for Medicare when you reach sixty-five or some time just before is quite easy. Call 1-800-633-4227 and you will be given instructions about how to apply. You can also apply by accessing the Medicare Web site at: www.medicare.gov. Several different plans are available. By calling older friends or relatives, you can decide on the plan that best fits your needs. It is wise too, if you can afford it, to pay for supplemental insurance, such as Blue Cross or Blue Shield. This way you can go to any doctor and not be locked into an HMO. AARP also has health plans that work well for some seniors. *Be aware that if you sign up for an HMO paid for by Medicare, you will be greatly restricted in your choice of physicians.* Outside specialists will not be allowed without appeals or the help of an attorney. You do usually get what you pay for in medicine as elsewhere.

Medicare has two parts: Part A and Part B. Part A provides for hospital coverage and some nursing home care. Part B is for doctors' office visits and some "durable medical equipment", such as walkers or wheelchairs. If you need assistance in deciding which insurance to use you can call the Health Insurance Counseling and Advocacy Program at 1-800-434-0222. Volunteers will be available to answer your questions. Now that there is a new Medicare law, questions are answered at the Web site, www.medicarerights.org. There is also another site: www.medicareinteractive.org. The new legislations appear to try and force seniors into HMOs. *This benefits the insurance companies, not the patients.* The new legislation is complicated, so no change should be made in your coverage until some careful research is done. Sticking with what you have, if it is working for you, is probably the best advice. Advocates are particularly important for some seniors.

> One ninety-four-year-old woman was having hip pain and saw an orthopedic surgeon. He took X-rays and immediately wanted to operate. He actually admitted, "I'm in the business of surgery." The woman's daughter insisted that another doctor be seen. This orthopedist said there was arthritis in the knees. After draining the knees, some medication was injected and the problem was resolved without surgery.

87. **All billing for Medicare and insurance is based on codes for procedures.** There are specific numbers for each procedure and if a doctor's office gives the wrong one to a lab or other facility, a bill may not be paid.

> A seventy-year-old-woman, who had Medicare and Blue Shield, had a routine Pap smear done by a board-certified gynecologist. She knew that Medicare authorized routine Pap smears every four years. To her dismay, she received a bill for $92.00 from the laboratory to which the Pap smear had been sent. On calling the lab, she discovered that the doctor's office had coded the bill as a diagnostic test, not a routine

one. The secretary at the doctor's office said they were in error and the lab would be called.

Thus, it is important to check the code the doctor's office used, if a bill is denied. Computers can make errors, or the individual putting the information into the computer may be having a bad day and make a mistake.

88. **If Medicare denies a claim for a doctor's visit, lab test, or procedure or there is a problem, an independent review process is possible by contacting Medicare Mediation at 1-800-841-1602 or by e-mail at: mediation@cagio.sdps.org.**

Important Terms for Seniors to Know

Medigap Insurance-Additional private insurance to cover medical costs above what Medicare will pay. AARP, Blue Shield, and others have these policies.

Boutique Medicine-Many doctors are charging an annual fee for patients to continue seeing them. (The fee ranges from one thousand to several thousand dollars a year.) In addition, most doctors will not bill Medicare or insurance companies and insist on being paid in cash for each visit.

Hospitalist-This is a doctor who is employed by the hospital and sees only in-patients. He or she has no outside practice and there is no contact with outside physicians. There is also no continuity of care, once a patient is discharged.

Respite Services-Short-term care or other services provided by outside agencies to care for an individual in need when the primary caretaker needs a break.

Personal emergency device-Offered by private companies to provide a way for emergency personnel to be contacted, if an elderly person needs emergency care, as with a fall or heart attack.

Dementia-A lessening of mental functions.

ADL-Activities of daily living- Occupational therapists help train or retrain patients in these activities after a stroke, injury, or other incapacitating disorder.

Healthcare proxy-A legal document that allows a family member, attorney, or other individual to make medical decisions about an individual.

Long-term care facility-This may be a nursing home or other facility that provides twenty-four-hour care for individuals who require this.

Durable power of attorney-This gives someone the right to make legal and other decisions for someone who no longer has the capacity to do so.

DNR-Do not resuscitate.

CHAPTER SIXTEEN

Overseas Health Care

Traveling overseas can be a wonderful experience unless medical problems develop. Then it can be a disaster, if some pre-trip preparation has not been done and information not obtained about good medical services and hospitals.

89. **If you might need health care overseas, it is best to try and obtain the names of reputable doctors or hospitals in the countries or places you are going to visit, *before* you leave on your trip**. Hotels usually have a doctor they can call but these may or may not be the best. It will pay to do research ahead of time by talking to your doctor or friends who travel.

90. **Be sure you don't start a new medication the day before or the day of a trip.**

> A physician was flying to San Francisco from New York when there was an emergency call for a doctor. She responded to the call and was directed to a large, older man who was gray and gasping for breath. The doctor immediately asked that his seat be reclined, so she could get a good look at him. On checking his blood pressure, she found it to be abnormally low. The man's wife said her husband's doctor in New York had prescribed a new blood pressure medicine the day before. Her husband, she said, had had high blood pressure for a long time. Several different medications had been tried before this new prescription was given. Fortunately, the plane was

about to land in San Francisco, so the physician asked that an ambulance meet the airplane. She gave the couple the name of her internist in San Francisco and her card. Later, a lovely note was received from the wife saying her husband was recovering and they were very grateful for her help. They had decided to change physicians when they returned home.

If a problem occurs during a flight, the pilots can call and speak with emergency room physicians via a program called Medlink. This is important because airplanes carry only a few drugs, oxygen, and sometimes defibrillators. Most physicians who are not general practitioners or family doctors are not comfortable or able to treat a wide variety of problems and may need advice from an ER physician.

91. **Most health insurance plans do not cover medical care outside the United States.** Those that do require you to call within forty-eight hours of receiving overseas medical care. If your health plan covers you for overseas care, be sure to save the receipts for any money you have paid for services. Medicare will not cover you unless you purchase a special Medi-gap policy. Information about obtaining this type of policy can be obtained from Medicare at 1-800-633-4227.

92. **Travel medical insurance can be purchased which may cover up to $50,000 depending on your age and what you pay for the policy.** The web site at: www.InsureMyTrip.com gives comparisons of different policies and rates. It is important to read the fine print of any insurance you decide to buy. There may be exclusion clauses that would make the insurance worthless for you. You can buy a policy for both a short stay or a long one.

93. **If you are working for a large U.S. company overseas, it is important to check about health care coverage,**

emergency medical care, and transportation for emergency medical care back to the United States. If a serious medical problem occurs, some large companies pay for air ambulance service back to the U.S. There are doctor groups that provide emergency medical care on flights back to the U.S. for big overseas companies. These groups contract with the big companies that send employees overseas. There are special companies that handle insurance for medical evacuation. International SOS is one, as is Global Travel Medical.

> Jim, a forty-year-old executive with a large American corporation accepted a position in the company's offices in Asia. He was allowed to take his family because it was a two-year assignment. The first few months were a time of discovering new friends, new foods, and new sights. Then tragedy struck. What had seemed like a common cold quickly developed into an ascending paralysis, which was finally diagnosed as Guillian-Barre syndrome. (In Asia, there is a severe form of this disorder that is often fatal). As the paralysis started to creep up his body, his wife and kids became panicked. Fortunately, Jim's father-in-law was a physician. He was called and immediately flew to his son-in-law's aid. An air ambulance was arranged and Jim was flown back to the United States. The best specialists were found and eventually Jim regained the ability to walk with crutches. His medical bills were at long last paid by the corporation for whom he worked.

CHAPTER SEVENTEEN

Alternative Medicine and Complementary Medicine

Traditional medicine has become so expensive and often of such poor quality that many are turning to alternative treatments. Some is good and some can be life-threatening. There are several different schools of alternative medicine: homeopathic, neuropathic, chiropractic, and traditional Chinese medicine. There are some unusual ones such as: Ayurveda medicine from India, Reiki from Japan, and Qi gong, a form of traditional Chinese medicine.

94. **Health food supplements or pills are not reviewed by the Food and Drug Administration, so be sure you know what they contain before buying or taking them.** It is much safer to stick with the well-known brands of vitamins and medicines approved by the FDA that you can buy in a drug store.

> Ralph, was taking sixty-five "natural medicines." His doctor found this out and ordered him to stop. Fortunately, the doctor took a good history because otherwise he would have had no way of knowing what the man was doing to his body. The hospital pharmacist visited Ralph while he was in the intensive care unit and also told him of the harm he was doing to himself.

Herbal medicines are not reviewed by the FDA and may contain unhealthy or dangerous substances. Many herbal medicines and supplements have serious interactions with prescription and non-prescription drugs. Most do not list all the ingredients on the labels. *Children should never be given herbal medicines.* Deaths have been documented following the ingestion of these by children. There have also been reports of herbal medicines interacting with standard medications and causing severe reactions. Thus, it is wise to check with your physician, if you plan on taking any herbal medicines.

95. **Acupuncture and massage may both be helpful with some medical problems**. It is important to be sure that the individuals treating you are licensed by the state because there are many unlicensed individuals who offer non-traditional medicine. If individuals are not licensed, use them at your own risk. There are good acupuncturists who are also M.D.s and some insurance companies will pay for their services.

Complementary Medicine

This is medicine or treatment that is used along with traditional medicine.

Massage, acupuncture are two good examples and both may be helpful for some problems.

CHAPTER EIGHTEEN

Long-Term Care

Long-term care is becoming more and more necessary, as individuals are living longer and longer. Those who can afford long-term care insurance are well advised to carry it.

96. **Nursing homes, assisted living facilities, and long-term care facilities vary from o.k. to bad.** By buying long-term care insurance, you can make sure you will not be put into a several bed ward or bankrupt your children or relatives. It is wise to check with your insurance agent about what the best long-term care insurance is for your pocket book. There are many different choices. Some have small deductibles and others have high deductibles. There are differences too, in the number of days covered. Read any policy carefully and ask lots of questions, so you will have a clear understanding of what is covered. To get the best medical care in your senior years, you need the best insurance possible. Good insurance is very much part of getting good medical care these days. Medicare will pay for care in some facilities for a limited number of days. However, private rooms may not be covered, so an individual would have one or more roommates.

There are no established standards, state, or federal regulations for **Assisted Living Facilities**. Many are very expensive and yet do not offer needed care. Thus much research should be done before paying for this type of care. The good assisted living facilities offer independence and security while providing meals and transportation. Medicare doesn't cover assisted living facilities, but some accept Medicaid; most do not. Some of these are called "residential care" facilities. For more information, you can call the National Center for Assisted Living at 1-202-842-4444 or view their Web site at: www.ncal.org.

Skilled Nursing Facility (SNF) is another name for a nursing home. A SNF should have a P.T., O.T., and M.D. on call. These facilities are subject to state and federal regulations. The Web site for the Assisted Living Federation is at: www.alfa.org and their telephone number is 1-703-691-8100. The Medicare Web site has a nursing home comparison site which is www.medicare.com.

If care is sought for yourself or a relative, the place to start is a visit to the facility. A great deal can be learned by walking in the door. Is it comfortable, clean, and welcoming? Are the residents dressed and clean, and do they seem comfortable? What is the quality of the food? Are the staff members pleasant, clean, and eager to help? What are the credentials of the medical personnel who care for the residents? Is the facility accredited and how long has it been in business? Who owns the facility and what are the initial and monthly charges? What is the ratio of staff members to residents?

97. **Individuals with limited financial resources can put their remaining sources of income or property into a trust for their children or relatives.** This way nursing home care will be paid for by Medicare or state welfare. However, then a private room is usually not an option and the medical and nursing care may not be the best.

It is important that a family member check every few days, if possible, to be sure that good medical and nursing care are being provided. Often, attending doctors make very few visits to nursing homes and the staff may be shorthanded. A lot can go by the wayside. Glasses, dental plates, clothes, and small items frequently disappear and have to be replaced.

A retired school teacher had a stroke and after several days in a hospital was transferred to a nursing home. She had a daughter who lived about twenty minutes away, but the daughter visited her mother infrequently. Fortunately, a good friend and her children visited often. On one visit, the teacher was found lying in bed at eleven o'clock in the morning. She told the friend that she had had no physical therapy or been allowed up in a wheelchair, as her doctor had ordered. The friend spoke with the head nurse and the director of the nursing home. On subsequent visits, the teacher said she was being given daily physical therapy, dressed, and allowed to be in a wheelchair. It made the difference in her recovery and her life.

CHAPTER NINETEEN

Home Health Care

Home health care can make the difference in a patient's life after a medical or surgical procedure. Patients are being sent home from the hospital after stays that are usually much too short. This way, more money is available for shareholders or CEOs.

98. Home health aides will be paid for by some insurance policies, Medicare, HMOs, and state programs. However, a doctor's prescription is needed for this to happen. Aides can take care of a patient's personal needs and some will shop for groceries and cook meals. It is important to check that the home health care agency is approved by Medicare. That way the agency must meet certain standards.

99. Good hospital care necessitates that the discharging physician make plans for the post-hospital care. The doctor's office can phone or fax the order for a home health aide. This must be done before a patient leaves the hospital. The order for a home health aide must be written by the patient's physician as part of his or her discharge orders. Aides are usually obtained from private companies that contract with the state, insurance companies, or HMOs. You can arrange and pay for your own aide, but without a doctor's prescription, the cost will not be covered by the state, your insurance, or an HMO.

When a patient leaves the hospital, it is the attending doctor's responsibility to write discharge orders. These are very important. They list any medications the patient is to take home, what post-hospital care is required, and orders for a home health aide, physical therapist, or occupational therapist, if they are needed. Most hospitals have a discharge coordinator who meets with the patient before he or she leaves the hospital. If a patient is being transferred to a nursing home or rehabilitation unit, this must be clearly stated in the doctor's orders. Arrangements for this then will be made by the nursing staff or other hospital personnel. If adequate planning is not done, serious problems can occur.

> An eighty-year-old woman, who lived alone, was hospitalized for heart failure. After she received several days of treatment in a local hospital, she had recovered enough to be sent home. No arrangements were made for her post-hospital care. Apparently, no one bothered to check that she lived alone and had few neighbors or relatives to help her. The woman tried to cope with day-to-day living but after two days, a neighbor found her lying on the kitchen floor in great pain. The elderly woman had fallen and broken her hip. She had to be taken back to the hospital for surgery and then had to have weeks of care in a rehabilitation hospital. This second hospitalization could very likely been avoided, if adequate post-hospital care arrangements had been made when she was discharged following the first hospitalization.

100. **Physical therapy and occupational therapy will be covered by some insurance plans, HMOs, and state programs with a prescription from your doctor.** Physical therapists and occupational therapists will make home visits after surgical procedures and for some medical problems. They can make a great difference in recovery from an orthopedic or other procedure.

CHAPTER TWENTY

Rehabilitation Care

Good rehabilitative care following surgery or a severe illness can make a dramatic difference in a patient's life. Physical therapists and occupational therapists are extremely important to a patient's recovery after orthopedic surgery or a severe illness. If orthopedic surgery is done on a come and go basis, plans and appointments for physical therapy should be made prior to the surgery.

101. **Care can be provided in a rehabilitation unit for varying periods, depending on your insurance coverage, HMO plan, Medicare, or state benefit**s. A doctor's orders are needed a*nd the physician in charge of your case should visit you frequently in the rehab unit.* Many surgeons are excellent technicians in the operating room, but leave the post-op care in a rehab unit to aides, nurses, or doctors-in-training. Major problems can then be overlooked. If a family member is in a rehab unit and not seen daily by a physician, it would be important to make a call to the doctor who is in charge. If your call does not produce better care, the next step would be to call the CEO or medical director of the hospital.

A physician visited an eighty-year-old neighbor in a rehab unit following his hip surgery. She was upset to hear him say that no doctor had seen him since his admission, two days before. She knew his internist and immediately called the doctor. This physician called the operating orthopedic surgeon and daily visits were then made by the orthopedist or one of his partners.

Physical therapy and occupational therapy should be available in all rehab units, if it is needed. All care needs to be monitored to be sure the proper orders have been written by the physician-in-charge and the needed care given. Also, arrangements need to be made for the post-op care, prior to the surgery. Meeting with the therapists before surgery is wise, as is asking your doctor about what plans, he or she has made for your post-op care.

One man had hand surgery but his doctor didn't make immediate plans for post-op therapy by the hand therapist. Thus, it took more therapy than should have been required. While she worked on his hand, the therapist told him several horror stories of patients whose hands had become almost fixed after hand surgery. She said she couldn't emphasize enough the need for immediate hand therapy after surgery. She said plans should be made with the therapist prior to any surgery.

WHICH MEDICAL PROFESSIONAL
WOULD YOU CHOOSE?

1.   A sixty-five-year-old man has pain and swelling in his right knee. He saw his internist who inserted a needle into the knee and took out fluid. No infection was reported. The doctor should refer him to a:

1. Sports medicine doctor

2. Cancer specialist

3. Physical therapist

4. Orthopedic surgeon

5. Rheumatologist

The answer is #4, an orthopedic surgeon. Problems involving the bones and joints should be seen by an orthopedic surgeon. In this case, referral was made to a physical therapist, who was wise enough to say she wasn't the appropriate referral.

****

2.   A fifty-year-old busy, much sought-after attorney, saw her physician for recurrent constipation and diarrhea. He told her she should take a stool softener. Soon, the attorney began to have abdominal pain. The woman called the physician, who said the pain went along with her irritable bowel syndrome. The woman knew she was in trouble and called the physician father of a good friend. He referred her to a:

1. General surgeon

2. Gynecologist

3. Gastroenterologist

4. Psychiatrist

5. Cancer specialist (Oncologist)

The appropriate referral was # 3, a gastroenterologist. The doctor did a colonoscopy and found a small, malignant polyp.

****

3.   A three-year-old boy had the sudden onset of his left eye deviating to the side. An eye doctor advised surgery. When the boy developed weakness of one side of his face, the parents sought a second opinion from another eye doctor. He referred the parents to:

1. Optometrist for eye exercises

2. Neurosurgeon

3. Neurologist

4. Optician

5. Radiologist

Once the child developed facial weakness, the appropriate referral was #3. The neurologist ordered an MRI, and a treatable brain tumor was found. It was surgically removed.

****

4.   A forty-five-year-old woman moved from California to New Orleans. She tried to do a lot of the moving herself and began to have extreme pain in her right shoulder. An internist referred her to a:

1. Orthopedic surgeon

2. Chiropractor

3. Physical therapist

4. Acupuncturist

5. Neurologist

The referral was appropriately to # 1, an orthopedic surgeon. The doctor found a "frozen shoulder" and advised physical therapy several times a week.

****

5.   A sixty-year-old, recently widowed man began to lose weight and was not eating well. His general doctor referred him to a:

1. Psychologist for counseling

2. Grief group

3. Radiologist

4. Gastroenterologist

5. Cancer specialist

The G.P. referred him to #4, a gastroenterologist. This doctor did numerous tests and found a large, cancerous mass in the bowel, Surgery and chemotherapy were advised. (It is always important to look for medical reasons for symptoms before assuming they are caused by an emotional or mental problem.)

****

6.   An eight-month-old baby girl was bright and alert, but still not rolling over or sitting. The pediatrician thought she was just taking her time. The grandmother insisted the baby should be checked by a:

1. Developmental pediatrician

2. Neurologist

3. Orthopedic surgeon

4. Another pediatrician

5. Pediatric neuromuscular specialist

The grandmother was a physician and knew that the appropriate referral was # 5, a pediatric neuromuscular specialist. Muscle diseases in children are given little emphasis in medical schools and even in training programs for neurologists.

****

7. A two-year-old little girl was not talking, but otherwise seemed fine. Her pediatrician referred her to:

    1. A speech therapist

    2. Developmental pediatrician

    3. Pediatric hearing center

    4. Child psychiatrist

    5. Ear-nose- throat doctor

The appropriate referral was to a pediatric hearing center, #3. The child's hearing was found to be poor and a referral to an ear, nose, and throat doctor was advised.

****

8. A three-year-old girl began limping on her right leg one day. Her parents looked at her legs and found a swollen, hot right knee. They immediately took the child to her pediatrician. He referred her to:

1. Orthopedist

2. Physical therapist

3. Rheumatologist

4. Laboratory

5. Ophthalmologist

The answer is #3, a rheumatologist. Because there was no history of injury, the pediatrician suspected juvenile rheumatoid arthritis (JRA). This occurs more frequently in little girls and starts usually in a single joint. The pediatric rheumatologist agreed with the diagnosis and referred the parents first to a laboratory for blood tests and then to a pediatric eye doctor for a slit-lamp examination. This referral was important because lab results may be negative, but a slit-lamp exam can show eye changes compatible with JRA.

****

9. A twenty-year-old became quite ill with a spiking, up and down, fever that went almost to 105 degrees. She also had pain on her right side. Her internist thought it was the "flu". However, when the fever persisted for three days, her physician father insisted she be referred to:

1. Infectious disease doctor

2. Ear-nose-throat doctor

3. Laboratory

4. Surgeon

5. Urologist

The correct answer is # 3, a laboratory. The father insisted a urine culture be done. (High spiking fevers and pain in the side indicate a kidney infection could be present.) There was a family history of kidney and urinary tract problems in the girl's family. The urine culture revealed a serious kidney infection. Once antibiotics were started, the fever subsided. Later X-rays of the kidneys revealed a congenital abnormality.

****

10.   A ten-year-old boy started going to the bathroom about every thirty minutes. His family doctor thought he was just anxious because the family were all high-achievers. The boy was bright and his parents expected him to always be at the top of his class. The doctor referred him to:

      1.   Child psychologist

      2.   Urologist

      3.   Laboratory

      4.   Radiologist

      5.   Child psychiatrist

The appropriate referral was to #2, a pediatric urologist. The doctor ordered kidney studies which revealed an enlarged, abnormal cystic kidney. Surgery was advised.

****

11.   A seventy-year-old male physician had a rapid, irregular heart beat. A cardiologist performed an angiogram, which entailed inserting a catheter into the right groin. A few days later the man developed severe pain and swelling in his right foot. His cardiologist was unavailable, so the physician referred himself to a:

1. Surgeon

2. Physical therapist

3. Orthopedic surgeon

4. Vascular surgeon

5. Radiologist

The correct answer is #3, an orthopedic surgeon. The patient was taken, at his insistence, to surgery and pus was found in a bone of the right foot. The infection was a result of the angiogram.

****

12.   A thirty-year-old, pregnant woman stopped at a stop sign and was suddenly hit in the rear by a large truck. She experienced severe neck and back pain. A physician friend urged her to immediately be seen by a:

1. Obstetrician

2. Orthopedic surgeon

3. Internist

4. Radiologist

5. Emergency room doctor

The appropriate referral was # 5, an emergency room doctor. Following a car accident, it is always advisable to be seen in an emergency room. X-rays can be taken and other studies performed as needed. Monitoring of the fetus should also be done. If necessary, the obstetrician and an orthopedic surgeon can be called.

****

13.   A two-week-old male infant had been taking the bottle well but then started having forceful vomiting. The parents were frightened and took the baby to their pediatrician. He referred them to a:

    1. Radiologist

    2. Pediatric gastroenterologist

    3. Pediatric surgeon

    4. Allergist

    5. Dietician

The pediatrician referred the parents to #3, a pediatric surgeon. The baby was found to have pyloric stenosis and did well after corrective surgery.

****

14.   A teenage girl hadn't had a period for several months. A gynecologist examined her and couldn't find a problem. She suggested the girl be referred to a:

    1. Endocrinologist

    2. Psychiatrist

    3. Family therapist

    4. Pediatrician

    5. Internist

The gynecologist referred the teenager to #2, a psychiatrist, who treated teens. The doctor suspected anorexia nervosa because there was also a marked weight loss.

****

15.   A teenage boy began limping and complaining of pain in his hip. His family doctor referred the youth to a:

1. Physical therapist

2. Radiologist

3. Orthopedic surgeon

4. Psychiatrist

5. Surgeon

The youth was referred to an orthopedic surgeon, #3. X-rays of the boy's hip revealed a condition called Legg-Perthe's disease.

****

16.   A fifty-year-old woman began to have popping and pain in her jaw. It became increasingly hard to open her jaw, to eat, or talk. In talking with her physician she said she had been under considerable stress because of a recent divorce and a long-distance move. The physician referred her to:

1. An ENT doctor

2. A dentist

3. Physical therapist

4. Occupational therapist

5. Masseur

The most appropriate referral would be # 5, a masseur. Stress is most often the cause of temporal-mandibular dysfunction or TMJ. There are exercises P.T.s can give that may be helpful, but the extra expenditure of money may increase stress, if dollars are a problem. Dentists and ENT doctors can be consulted, but reduction of stress by every means possible should be the primary goal.

HEALTH CARE STATISTICS

- In 2000, the World Health Organization ranked health care in the United States at number thirty-seven.

- The United States ranks twentieth or lower as compared in other developed nations as to life expectancy, infant mortality, and immunizations.

- The healthiest twenty percent of Americans spend about $14 each year on health care.

- The number of uninsured in the U.S. is about 43 million individuals. (46 million in 2006).

- The administrative costs for health care in the U.S. are estimated at 25 to 50 percent.

- Medicare recipients use 42 percent of the drugs purchased in the U.S.

- The pharmaceutical companies made $38 billion dollars in profits in 2000.

- 45 to 50 percent of personal bankruptcies are due to medical bills.

- Ten percent of the population accounts for 70 percent of health care costs.

- Cutting the medical administrative costs in half would save $200 billion dollars a year as of 2002.

- Drug companies spend about three times as much on marketing and advertising as on research and development.

- Drug companies have the highest profit margin of all American corporations.

- Drug prices are bout 60 percent higher than in the United Kingdom and Canada.

(Ref: *Health Care Meltdown* by Robert LeBow, M.D.)

More Statistics

* Generic drugs save an average of $45.50 for every prescription sold.

* For every one percent increased use of generic drugs, consumers could save 1.3 billion dollars.

* Currently, generic drugs save consumers $56.7 billion dollars each year.

(Ref: Buehler, G. (Director FDA Office of Generic Drugs)

---

* Healthcare insurance carriers reject 30 percent of all claims submitted.

* Forty-three percent of health-care lobbyists are former members of Congress.

* Percent of revenue spent by drug companies on marketing and administration is 30 percent.

* Amount spent on lobbying in Washington D.C. by pharmaceutical companies in 2003 was $143 million.

* National Institute of Health budget for 2005 was $27.9 billion.

* Americans spent more than $200 billion for prescriptions in 2004.

(Ref: Stanford Medicine -Summer 2005)

HEALTH CARE FOR MILITARY PERSONNEL AND FAMILIES

In the past, military personnel and their families received their primary care from drop-in clinics and hospital emergency rooms. Patients were allowed to carry their own charts from doctor to doctor or military facility to facility. This now has changed. Instead, active-duty service personnel are automatically registered in the Defense Enrollment Eligibility Reporting System. (DEERS). This entitles service personnel to medical care in specified locations or offices. Medical records are transferred electronically from one facility to another. A private physician must have a contract with the armed services to be able to care for military personnel.

There are different levels of care under the Tricare plan:

- Tricare prime-functions like a PPO and costs an individual more.

- Standard-there may be a twenty percent cost to the individual.

- Tricare for Life-offers coverage to service personnel who are sixty-five and eligible for Medicare. It pays after Medicare, if the individual has purchased part B of Medicare.

Military dependents of active-duty personnel must enroll in DEERS to be eligible for Tricare benefits. Address changes, divorce, adoption or birth of a child, death, or retirement all necessitate that records be up-dated. The nearest place to register can be found at: www.dmdc.ord.mil. An 800 number can be called for information at: 1-800-538-9552. There are also Tricare offices in each region.

Helpful Numbers

Tricare West-	1-888-TRIWEST
Tricare North-	1-877-TRICARE
Tricare South-	1-800-444-5445
Tricare Prime Remote-	1-888-363-2273
Mail Order Pharmacy-	1-866-363-8667
Retiree Dental Plan-	1-888-838-8737
Tricare Dental Program-	1-800-866-8499
Tricare for Life-	1-866-773-0404
Senior Pharmacy Program-	1-877-363-6337

Tricare Overseas

Pacific-	1-888-777-8343
Europe-	1-888-777-8343
Canada/Latin America-	1- 888-777-8343
Puerto Rico/Virgin Islands-	1-888-777-8343

VETERANS HEALTH CARE

There have been many studies of the health care that veterans are and are not receiving. Mental health facilities are particularly lacking. It is estimated that fifty percent of homeless individuals are veterans with mental illness. Under the medical benefits plan, the basic services covered are:

- Outpatient medical, surgical, mental health and substance abuse.

- Inpatient hospital, medical, surgical, mental health and substance abuse.

- Prescription drugs and some over-the counter drugs, medical and surgical supplies in the Veterans' Administration formulary.

- Emergency care in Veterans' facilities.

- Emergency care in non-Veterans' facilities under some conditions.

- Rehabilitation services.

- Counseling.

- Durable medical equipment.

- Pregnancy and delivery.

- Hospice.

- Home health services.

Health Care for Reservists Who Have Been Mobilized Since September 2001.

In the past, National Guard and Reserve members could keep their health care coverage for no more than six months after they left active duty. Now they will be offered military health care coverage for as long as eight years after they return to civilian life. They will need to stay in the Reserves and the length of coverage will depend on how long they served and how long they plan to stay in the National Guard or Reserves.

Individual coverage will be $50 to $150 per month and family coverage will be $100 to $300 per month.

The Veteran's Health Administration web site is www.va.gov and their telephone number is 1-877-222-8387

HEALTH CARE FOR INDIVIDUALS WITH DISABILITES

Medicaid is a state-run program that was set up for individuals with low incomes or persons with disabilities. The federal government helps pay for Medicaid. Each state has different qualifications. In California the program is called Medi-Cal. Unfortunately, few California doctors accept Medi-Cal patients because the remuneration is very small or the program will not pay at all. The regulations constantly change, and it is an extremely poor program. The result is that many Medi-Cal patients in California use emergency rooms as their primary source of medical care. This allows for no continuity of care and makes the cost of patient care extremely high. Some low-income patients are eligible for both Medicare and Medicaid. Information about eligibility can be obtained from the local social service or welfare office. The rules are complex, but, in general, low income individuals who are blind, disabled, or elderly should qualify. Teenagers who are living on their own with little income can also apply.

STATE MEDICAL BOARDS

Alabama

Board of Medical Examiners
(334) 242-4116
Fax: (334) 242-4155

Alaska

State Medical Board
(907) 269-8160
Fax: (907) 269-8156

Arizona

State Medical Board
(602) 255-3751
Fax: (602) 255 1848

Arkansas

State Medical Board
(501) 296-1802
Fax: (501) 296-1805

California

Medical Board
(800) 633-2322
Fax: (916) 263-2387

Colorado

Board of Medical Practice
(303) 894-7690
Fax: (303) 894-7692

Connecticut

Department of Public Health
(860) 509-7586
Fax: (860) 509-7553

Delaware

Board of Medical Practice
(302) 739-4522
Fax: (302) 739-2711

District of Columbia

Board of Medicine
(202) 727-5365
Fax: (202) 727-4087

Florida

Board of Medicine
(904) 488-0595
Fax: (904) 922-3040

Georgia

State Board of Medical Examiners
(404) 656-3913
Fax: (404) 656-9723

Hawaii

Board of Medical Examiners
(808) 586-2708
Fax: (808) 586-2689

Idaho

State Board of Medicine
(208) 334-2844
Fax: (208) 334-2801

Illinois

Department of Professional Regulation
Discipline: (312) 814-4500
Fax: (312) 814-1837
Licensure: (217) 785-0800
Fax: (217) 524-2169

Indiana

Health Professions Bureau
(317) 232-2960
Fax: (317) 233-4236

Iowa

State Board of Medical Examiners
(515) 281-5171
Fax: (515) 242-5908

Kansas

Board of Healing Arts
(913) 296-7413
Fax: (913) 296-0852

Kentucky

Board of Medical Licensure
(502) 429-8046
Fax: (520) 429-9923

Louisiana

State Board of Medical Examiners
(504) 524-6763
Fax: (504) 568-8893

Maine

Board of Licensure in Medicine
(207) 287-3601
Fax: (not listed)

Maryland

Board of Physician Quality Assurance
(800) 492-6836
Fax: (410) 764-2478

Massachusetts

Board of Registration in Medicine
(617) 727-3086
Fax: (617) 451-9568

Michigan

Board of Medicine

(517) 335-0918

Fax: (517) 373- 2179

Minnesota

Board of Medical Practice

(612) 617-2130

Fax: (612) 617-2186

Mississippi

State Board of Medical Licensure

(601) 354-6645

Fax: (602) 897-4159

Missouri

State Board of Registration for the Healing Arts

(573) 751-0098

Fax: (573) 751-3166

Montana

Board for Medical Examiners

(406) 444-4284

Fax: (406) 444-9396

Nebraska

Department of Health

(402) 471-2118

Fax: (402) 471-3577

Nevada

State Board of Medical Examiners

(702) 688-2559

Fax: (702) 688-2321

New Hampshire

Board of Medicine

(603) 271-1203

Fax: (603) 271-6702

New Jersey

State Board of Medical Examiners

(609) 826-7100

Fax: (609) 984-3930

New Mexico

State Board of Medical Examiners

(505) 827-5022

Fax: (505) 827-7377

New York

State Board of Medicine

(518) 474-3841

Fax: (518) 473- 0578

North Carolina

Medical Board

(919) 828-1212

Fax: (919) 828-1295

North Dakota

State Board of Medical Examiners

(701) 328-6500

Fax: (701) 328-6505

Ohio

State Medical Board

(614) 466-3934

Fax: (641) 728-5946

Oklahoma

Board of Medical Licensure and Supervision

(405) 848-6841

Fax: (405) 848-8240

Oregon

Board of Medical Examiners

(503) 229-5770

Fax: (503) 229-6543

Pennsylvania

State Board of Medicine

(717) 787-2381

Fax: (717) 787-7769

Rhode Island

Board of Medical Licensure and Discipline

(401) 277-3855

Fax: (401) 277-2158

South Carolina

Board of Medical Examiners

(803) 737-9300

Fax: (803) 737-9314

South Dakota

State Board of Medical and Osteopathic Examiners

(605) 334-8343

Fax: (605) 336-0272

Tennessee

Board of Medical Examiners

(615) 532-4384

Fax: (615) 532-5164

Texas

State Board of Medical Examiners

(800) 201-9353/ (512) 305-7010

Fax: (512) 305-7008

Utah

Department of Commerce/Division of Occupational and Professional Licensure

(801) 530-6628

Fax: (801) 530-6511

Vermont

Board of Medical Practice

(802) 828-2673

Fax: (802) 828-5450

Virginia

Board of Medicine
(804) 662-7005
Fax: (804) 558-2084

Washington

Medical Quality Assurance Commission
(360) 664-8480
Fax: (360) 586-4573

West Virginia

Board of Medicine
(304) 558-2921
Fax: (304) 558-2084

Wisconsin

Medical Examining Board
(608) 266-1188
Fax: (608) 267-0644

Wyoming

Board of Medicine
(307) 778-7053
Fax: (307) 778-2069

STATE INSURANCE OFFICES
AND RESOURCES

Alabama

Governor's Office
(334) 242-7100

Health Care Reform Task Force
(334) 613-5318

Department of Insurance
(334) 269-3550

Alabama Medicaid Agency
(334) 242-5600

Department of Health
(334) 613-5300

Alaska

Governor's Office
(907) 465-3500

Department of Health and Social Services
(907) 465-3030

Department of Commerce and Economic Development
(907) 465-2515

Division of Medical Assistance, Department of Health
Insurance
(907) 465-3355

Arizona

Governor's Office
(602) 542-4331

Department of Health Services
(602) 542-1025

Department of Insurance
(602) 912-8400

Arizona Health Care Cost Containment System
(602) 417-4000

Arkansas

Governor's Office
(501) 682-2345

Department of Health
(501) 681-2111

Department of Insurance
(501) 371-2600

Division of Medical Services, Department of Human
Services
(501) 682-8292

California

Governor's Office
(916) 445-5106

Department of Health Services/ Medi-Cal
(916) 657-0025

Department of Insurance
(916) 492-3500

California Public Employees Retirement System (CALPERS)
(916) 326-3991

Health Insurance Plan of California (HIPC)
(916) 786-7279

Colorado

Governor's Office
(303) 866-2471

Department of Social Services Health Plans and Medicaid
Services
(303) 866-6092

Department of Regulatory Agencies, Department of Insurance
(303) 894-7499

Office of Health Care Policy and Financing
(303) 866-2993

Department of Health
(303) 692-2000

Connecticut

Governor's Office
(860) 566-4840

Department of Public Health
(860) 509-8000

Department of Insurance
(860) 297-3800

Department of Social Services
(860) 424-5008

Office of Health Care Access
(860) 566-3880

Delaware

Governor's Office
(302) 739-4104

Department of Health and Social Services
(302) 577-4900

Department of Insurance
(302) 739- 4251

Department of Health and Social Services Medicaid Unit
(302) 577-4900

Delaware Health Care Commission
(302) 739-6907

Public Health Division
(302) 739-4701

District of Colombia

Office of the Mayor
(202) 727-2980

Department of Human Services
(202) 727-8500

Insurance Administration
(202) 727-8000 ext. 3007

Commission on Health Care
(202) 727-0735

Task Force on Health Care Reform
Office of Policy (202) 727-6979

D.C. Health Policy Council
(202) 727-9239

Florida

Governor's Office
(904) 388-2272

Department of Insurance
(904) 922-3100

Agency for Health Care Administration
(904) 488-3560

Health and Rehabilitative Services Department
(904) 488-9334

Department of Health
(904) 487-3220

Georgia

Governor's Office
(404) 656-1776

Health Planning Agency
(404) 656-0655

Department of Insurance
(404) 656-2056

Department of Medical Assistance
(404) 656-2515

Georgia Health Policy Center
(404) 651-3104

Governor's Commission on Health Care
(404) 657-4479

Division of Public Health
(404) 657-2700

Hawaii

Governor's Office
(808) 586-0034

Department of Health
(808) 586-4400

Commerce and Consumer Affairs Department, Insurance
Division
(808) 586-2790

Department of Human Services, Medicaid Division
(808) 586-5500

Idaho

Governor's Office
(208) 334-2100

Department of Health and Welfare
(208) 334-5747

Department of Insurance
(208) 334-4250

Illinois

Governor's Office
(217) 782-6830

Department of Public Health
(217) 782-5750

Department of Insurance
(217) 782-4515

Department of Public Aid
(217) 782-1214

Indiana

Governor's Office
(317) 232-4567

Department of Health
(317) 383-6100

Office of Medicaid Policy
(317) 232-2385

Department of Insurance and Planning
(317) 233-4448

Iowa

Governor's Office
(515) 281-5211

Department of Public Health
(515) 281-5787

Department of Commerce, Division of Insurance
(515) 281-5705

Department of Human Services, Division of Medical
Services
(515) 281-8621

Kansas

Governor's Office
(913) 296-3232

Legislative Liaison/ Health
(913) 296-6991

Department of Insurance
(913) 296-7801 or (913) 296-3071

SRS Division of Adult Medical Services
(913) 296-3133

SRS Division of Medicaid
(913) 296-3981

Department of Health and the Environment
(913) 296-1343

Kentucky

Governor's Office
(502) 564-2611

Department of Insurance
(502) 564-6027 or (800) 595-6053

Cabinet for Families and Children
(502) 564-7130

Department of Medicaid Services, Cabinet for Health
Services
(502) 564-4321

Louisiana

Governor's Office
(504) 342-7015

Louisiana Health Commission
(504) 342-5900

Department of Insurance
(504) 342-5900

Department of Health and Hospitals, Bureau of Health Services Financing

(504) 342-3891

Maine

Governor's Office
(207) 287-3531

Office of Policy and Legal Analysis
(207) 287-1670

Department of Human Services
(207) 287-3707

Bureau of Insurance
(207) 624-8475

Health Care Reform Commission
(207) 624-8655

Bureau of Medical Services, Department of Human Services
(207) 287-2674

Health Care Finance Commission
(207) 287-3006

Department of Mental Health
(207) 287-4200

Maryland

Governor's Office
(410) 974-3901

Department of Health
(410) 225-6505

Insurance Administration
(410) 468-2000 or (800) 468-2000

Health Care Access and Cost Commission
(410) 764-3460

Massachusetts

Governor's Office
(616) 727-6250

Joint Legislative Committee on Health Care
(617) 722-2130

Health and Human Services Executive Office
(617) 727-0077

Division of Medical Assistance
(617) 521-7794 or (617) 521-7777

Health Care Purchasing Group
(617) 270-4911

Michigan

Governor's Office
(517) 373-3400

Department of Community Health
(517) 335-8000

Department of Commerce, Insurance Bureau
(517) 373-9273

Department of Social Services, Medical Services
Administration
(517) 335-5001

Minnesota

Governor's Office
(612) 296-3391

Department of Health
(612) 623-5000

Department of Commerce
(612) 623-5000

Department of Human Services
(612) 296-6117

Health Care Commission
(612) 282-6374

Minnesota Health Data Institute
(612) 228-4370

Insurance Commission
(612) 296-7033

Mississippi

Governor's Office
(601) 359-3100

Department of Health
(601) 960-7400

Department of Insurance
(601) 359-3569

Division of Medicaid
(601) 359-6050

Missouri

Governor's Office
(314) 751- 3222

Joint Legislative Committee on Health Care Policy and Planning
(314) 751-2128

Department of Health
(314) 751-4126

Department of Insurance
(314) 751-6922

Department of Social Services, Division of Medical Services
(314) 751-6922

Department of Health, Bureau of Health Systems Research and Development
(314) 751-0693

Montana

Governor's Office
(406) 444-3111

Department of Insurance
(416) 444-2040

Health Care Advisory Committee
(406) 431-2770

Department of Public Health and Human Services
(406) 444-4540

Nebraska

Governor's Office
(402) 471-2244

Department of Health, Division of Health Policy
(402) 471-2337

Department of Insurance
(402) 471-9147

Interagency Health Care Commission
(402) 471-2256

Blue Ribbon Coalition on Health Care
(402) 397-0203

Nevada

Governor's Office
(702) 687-5670

Nevada State Health Division
(702) 687-4740

Division of Insurance
(702) 687-4270

Medicaid/ Welfare Division
(702) 687-4867

New Hampshire

Governor's Office
(603) 271-2121

Department of Health and Human Services
(603) 271-4685

Department of Insurance
(603) 271-4685

Department of Insurance
(603) 271-2261

Office of Medical Services
(603) 271-4353

New Jersey

Governor's Office
(609) 292-6000

Department of Health
(609) 292 7837

Department of Insurance
(609) 292-5363

Division of Medical Assistance and Health Services
(609) 588-2600

Health Access New Jersey
(609) 292-0098

Small Employer Health Benefits Program
(609) 633-1887

New Mexico

Governor's Office
(505) 827-2389

Department of Health, Division of Public Health
(505) 827-2389

Department of Insurance
(505) 827-4601

Department of Human Services, Medical Assistance Division
(505) 827-3106

Health Care Initiatives
(505) 827-7500

New York

Governor's Office
(518) 474-8390

Department of Social Services, Division of Health and Long Term Care
(518) 474-9132

Joint Legislative Council on Health Care Financing
(518) 455-2067

Office for the Aging
(518) 474-5731

Department of Insurance
(518) 474-6600 or (518) 474-4556

Department of Social Services
(518) 474-9132

Health and Hospital Corporation
(212) 788-3327

Department of Health-Medicaid Management
(518) 474-2482

North Carolina

Governor's Office
(919) 733-4240

Department of Health
(919) 733-4984

Department of Insurance
(919) 733-7349 or (919) 733-7343

Division of Medical Assistance
(919) 733-2060

Health Care Reform Commission
(919) 715-4740

State Health Plan Purchasing Alliance Board
(919) 715-4440

North Dakota

Governor's Office
(701) 328-2200

Department of Health
(701) 328-2372

Department of Insurance
(701) 328-2440

Department of Human Services, Medical Services
Division
(701) 328-2321

Ohio

Governor's Office
(614) 466-3555

Department of Health
(614) 466-2253

Department of Insurance
(614) 644-2658

Department of Human Services, Office of Medicaid
(614) 644-0140

Oklahoma

Governor's Office
(405) 521-2342

Department of Health
(405) 271-4200

Department of Insurance
(405) 521-2828

Oklahoma Health Care Authority
(405) 951-4700

Oklahoma Health Care Alliance
(405) 951-4700

Department of Human Services
(405) 521-2778

Oregon

Governor's Office
(503) 378-3111

Human Resources Department, Medical Assistance
(503) 378-2422

Department of Consumer and Business Services, Insurance Division
(503) 378-4271

Health Care Planning and Policy Committee
(503) 378-2422

Department of Insurance
(503) 521-2828 or (800) 542-3104

Pennsylvania

Governor's Office
(717) 787-2500

Department of Health
(717) 787-1783

Department of Insurance
(717) 787-5173

Department of Public Welfare, Office of Medical Assistance
(717) 787-1870

Rhode Island

Governor's Office
(401) 277-2080

Department of Health
(401) 277-2231

Insurance Division
(401) 277-2223

Department of Human Services, Division of Medical Services
(401) 464-2176

Rite Care
(401) 464-3113

South Carolina

Governor's Office
(803) 734-9818

Health and Environmental Control Department
(803) 734-4880

Department of Insurance
(803) 737-6160

State Department of Health and Human Services
(803) 253-6100

South Dakota

Governor's Office
(605) 773-3212

Department of Health
(605) 773-3361

Department of Social Services
(605) 773-3165

Department of Commerce and Regulation, Division of Insurance
(605) 773-4104

Commission on Insurance
(605) 773-3563

Tennessee

Governor's Office
(615) 741-2001

Department of Health
(615) 741-3111

Department of Commerce and Insurance
(615) 741-2241

Department of Health, TennCare Bureau
(615) 741-0213

Texas

Governor's Office
(512) 463-2000

Department of Health
(512) 458-7111

Department of Insurance
(512) 463-6464

Health and Human Services Commission
(512) 424-6500

Texas Insurance Purchasing Alliance
(512) 472-3956

Utah

Governor's Office
(801) 538-1000

Department of Health
(801) 538-6101

Department of Insurance
(801) 538-3800 D

Department of Health, Division of Health Care Planning
(801) 538-6406

Utah Health Policy Commission
(801) 538-6984

Vermont

Governor's Office
(802) 828-3333

Department of Health
(802) 863-7280

Division of Medicaid
(802) 241-2880

Department of Banking, Insurance and Securities
(802) 828-3301

Vermont Health Care Authority
(802) 828-2900

Virginia

Governor's Office
(804) 786-2211

Health Department
(804) 786-3561

Department of Medical Assistance Services
(804) 786-8099

State Corporation Commission, Bureau of Insurance
(804) 371-9694 or (800) 371-9694

Joint Commission on Health Care
(804) 786-5445

Washington

Governor's Office
(360) 753-6780

Health Department
(360) 586-5846

Insurance Department
(360) 753-7301

Department of Social and Health Services, Medical
Assistance Administration
(360) 753-1777

Washington Health Care Authority
(360) 923-2600

West Virginia

Governor's Office
(304) 558-2000

Health and Human Resources Department
(304) 926-1700

Department of Insurance
(304) 558-3386 or (304) 558-3394

Health Care Cost Review Authority
(304) 558-7000

West Virginia Health Care Reform
(304) 558-0530

Center for Rural Health Development
(304) 344-4471

Office of Medicaid Services, Department of Health and
Human Services
(304) 926-1700

Wisconsin

Governor's Office
(608) 266-1212

Insurance Commission
(608) 266-0102

Department of Health and Social Services Bureau of Health
Care Financing
(608) 266-2522

Wyoming

Governor's Office
(307) 777-7434

Department of Health
(307) 777-7656

Department of Insurance
(307) 777-7401

Division of Health Care Financing
(307) 777-7531

Wyoming Health Resources Network
(307) 635-2930

Note: This information was kindly provided by *Patients are Powerful*. Their web site is www.patientsarepowerful.org and they can be contacted at (916)-652-2293.

MEDICAL RESOURCES FOR SPECIAL NEEDS KIDS

Alaska

Health Care Program for Children with Special Needs
1211 Gambell Street
Suite 30
Anchorage, AK 99501
(907) 272-1534

American Samoa

Maternal & Child Health & Crippled Children's Program
LBJ Tropical Medical Center
Division of Public Health
Pago Pago, American Samoa 96799
011 (684) 633-4606

Arkansas

Children's Medical Services
Department of Human Services
P.O. Box 1437, slot #526
Little Rock, AR 72203
(501) 682-2277
(800) 482-5850 (in Arkansas)

California

Children's Medical Services Branch
714 P Street, Room #350
Sacramento, CA 95814
(916) 654-0499

Colorado

Health Care Program for Children with Special Needs
Colorado Department of Health
4300 Cherry Creek Drive South
Denver, CO 80222
(303) 692-2370

Connecticut

Children with Special Health Care Needs
Department of Health
999 Asylum Avenue
Hartford, CT 06106
(203) 566-3994

District of Colombia

Health Services for Children with Special Needs
State Department of Human Services
19th and Massachusetts Avenue S.E.
Washington, DC 20003
(202) 675-5214

Florida

Children's Medical Services Program
Department of Health and Rehabilitation Services
1317 Winewood Boulevard
Building B, Room #128
Tallahassee, FL 32399
(904) 487-2690

Georgia

Children's Medical Services
Department of Human Resources
2600 Skyland Drive N.E.
Atlanta, GA 30319
(404) 679-2126

Idaho

Children's Special Health Program
Department of Health and Welfare
P.O. Box 83720, 4th Floor
Boise, ID 83720
(208) 334-3940

Illinois

Division of Specialized Care for Children
2815 W. Washington, Suite #300
Springfield, IL 62794
(217) 793-2350

Indiana

Children's Special Health Care Services
Indiana State Department of Health
1330 W. Michigan
P.O. Box 1964
Indianapolis, IN 46206
(317) 383-6273

Iowa

Child Health Specialty Clinic
University of Iowa
247 Hospital School
Iowa City, IA 52242
(319) 356-1469

Kansas

Services for Children with Special Health Care Needs
State Department of Health and Environment
900 S.W. Jackson, Room #1005-N
Topeka, KS 66612
(913) 296-1313

Kentucky

Commission for Children with Special Health Care Needs
982 Eastern Parkway
Louisville, KY 40217
(502) 595-3264

Louisiana

Children's Special Health Services
Department of Health and Hospitals
Office of Public Health
P.O. Box 60630
Room #607
New Orleans, LA 70160
(504) 568-5055

Maine

Bureau of Children with Special Needs
Department of Mental Health and Mental Retardation
State House, Station #40
Augusta, ME 04333
(207) 287-4250

Maryland

Children's Medical Services
Department of Mental Health
201 W. Preston Street, 4th Floor
Baltimore, MD 21201
(410) 225-5580

Massachusetts

Division for Children with Special Health Needs
Bureau of Family and Community Health
150 Tremont Street
Boston, MA 02111
(617) 727-3372

Michigan

Children's Special Health Care Services
Department of Public Health
3423 N. Martin Luther King Boulevard
P.O. Box 30195
Lansing, MI 48909
(517) 335-8961

Minnesota

Minnesota Children with Special Health Needs
Division of Family Services
Department of Health
717 Delaware Street S.E.
P.O. Box 9441
Minneapolis, MN 55440
(612) 623-5150

Missouri

Bureau of Special Health Care Needs
Department of Health
P.O. Box 570
Jefferson City, MO 65102
(314) 751-6246

Montana

Children with Special Health Needs
Bureau of Maternal and Child Health
1400 Broadway, Room #314
Helena, MT 59620
(406) 444-4740

Nebraska

Medically Handicapped Children's Program
Department of Social Services
301 Centennial Mall South
Lincoln, NE 68509
(402) 471-3121

New Hampshire

Bureau of Special Medical Services
Office of Family and Community Health
Division of Public Health Services
6 Hazen Drive
Concord, NH 03301
(603) 271-4499
(800) 852-3345 (in New Hampshire)

New Jersey

Special Child Health Services
Department of Health, CN 634
Trenton, NJ 08625
(609) 292-5676

New Mexico

Children's Medical Services
State Department of Health
P.O. Box 968
Santa Fe, NM 87502
(595) 827-2574

New York

Physically Handicapped Children's Services
Bureau of Child and Adolescent Health
Corning Tower Bldg., Room 208
Empire State Plaza
Albany, NY 12237
(518) 474-2001

North Carolina

Children's Special Health Services
Department of Environment, Health, and Natural Resources
P.O. Box 27687
Raleigh, NC 27611
(919) 733-7437

North Dakota

Children's Special Health Services
Department of Human Services
State Capitol
600 E. Boulevard Avenue
Bismarck, ND 58505
(701) 328-2436

Oklahoma

Special Health Care Needs Unit
Oklahoma Health Care Authority
Lincoln Plaza, Suite 124
4545 No. Lincoln Boulevard
Oklahoma City, OK 73105
(405) 530-3400

Pennsylvania

Division of Children's Special Health Care Needs
Bureau of Maternal and Child Preventative Health
State Department of Health
P.O. Box 90, Room #714
Harrisburg, PA 17108
(800) 852-4453

Puerto Rico

Crippled Children's Services
125 Diego Avenue
Puerto Nuevo, PR 00921
(809) 781-2728

Rhode Island

Office of Special Needs
Department of Education
Roger Williams Bldg., Rm. 209
22 Hayes Street
Providence, RI 02908
(401) 444-5685

South Carolina

Children's Rehabilitative Services
Division of Children's Health
Department of Health and Environment Control
2600 Bull Street
Columbia, SC 29201
(803) 737-0465

South Dakota

Children's Special Health Services
Department of Health
445 E. Capital
Pierre, SD 57501
(605) 773-3737

Tennessee

Children's Special Services
Department of Health
Tennessee Tower, 11th floor
312 Eighth Avenue North
Nashville, TN 37247
(615) 741-8530

Texas

Children's Health Division
Texas Department of Health
1100 W. 49th Street
Austin, TX 78756
(512) 458-7355

Utah

Children with Special Health Care Needs, Community and
Family Health Services
Utah Department of Health
44 N. Medical Drive
Salt Lake City, UT 84114
(801) 584-8284

Vermont

Children with Special Health Care Needs
Department of Health
108 Cherry St.
Burlington, VT 05401
(802) 863-7338

(U.S.) Virgin Islands

Services for Children with Special Health Care Needs
Division of Maternal and Child Health
Department of Health
3200 Estate Richmond
Christiansted
St. Croix, VI 00820
(809) 773-1311

Virginia

Children's Specialty Services
Virginia Department of Health
1500 E. Main Street, Suite #135
Richmond, VA 23219
(804) 864-7706

Washington

Children with Special Health Care Needs
P.O. Box 47880
Olympia, WA 98504
(360) 753-0908

West Virginia

Handicapped Children's Services
Office of Maternal and Child Health
Bureau of Public Health
1116 Quarrier Street
Charleston, WV 25301
(304) 558-5388

Wisconsin

Program for Children with Special Health Care Needs
Department of Health and Social Services
1414 E. Washington Avenue, Room #167
Madison, WI 53703
(608) 266-7826

Wyoming

Children's Health Services
Hathaway Office Bldg., Room #462
Cheyenne, WY 82002
(307) 777-7941

Note: This information was taken from the author's book *Raising a Handicapped Child*, Oxford University Press (2000)

NATIONAL TOLL-FREE
TELEPHONE NUMBERS

Toll-Free Directory Assistance	1-800-555-1212
AIDS Hotline	1-800-342-2437
AMC Cancer Information Center	1-800-525-3777
American Council of the Blind	1-800-424-8666
American Kidney Fund	1-800-638-8299
American Speech-Language Association	1-800-638-8255
Better Hearing Institute	1-800-327-9355
Cancer Information Service	1-800-422-6237
Epilepsy Information Line	1-800-257-1227
International Hearing Society	1-800-521-5247
International Shriners Headquarters	1-800-237-5055
Juvenile Diabetes Foundation.	1-800-223-1138
Lung Line Information Service	1-800-222-5864
National Center for Stuttering	1-800-221-2483
National Cystic Fibrosis Foundation	1-800-344-4823
National Down Syndrome Congress	1-800-232-6372

National Down Syndrome Society	1-800-221-4602
National Easter Seal Society	1-800-221-6827
National Health Information Center	1-800-336-4797
Referral Service National Library Service for the Blind & Physically Handicapped	1-800-424-8567
National Protection & Advocacy	1-800-776-5746
National Spinal Cord Injury Hotline	1-800-526-3456
National SIDS Foundation	1-800-221-7437
Orton Dyslexia Society	1-800-222-3123
Prevent Blindness America	1-800-221-3004
RP Foundation Fighting Blindness	1-800-683-5555
Special Needs Network	1-800-471-0026
Spina Bifida Association for America	1-800-621-3141
Alzheimer's Association	1-800-272-3900
Arthritis Foundation	1-800-238-7800
Asthma information	1-800-822-2762
Autism Society	1-800-328-8476
American Brain Tumor Association	1-800-886-2282
American Cancer Society Information	1-800-227-2345
AIDS Treatment Information Service	1-800-448-0440

Alcohol and Drug Helpline	1-800-821-4357
Food Allergy Network	1-800-929-4040
National Center for Alternative Medicine	1-888-644-6226
American Podiatric Association	1-800-366-8227

STATE INSURANCE REGULATORS

Alabama

Department of Public Health
Division of Managed Care Compliance
RSA Tower, Suite #750
P.O. Box 303017
Montgomery, AL 36130-3017
(334) 206-5366

Alaska

Division of Insurance
3601 C Street, Suite #1324
Anchorage, AK 99503-5948
(907) 269-7900

Consumer Services
(800) 467-8725

Arizona

Department of Insurance
2910 N 44th Street, Suite #210
Phoenix, AZ 85018
(602) 912-8444

Consumer Assistance Division
(800) 325-2548

Arkansas

Arkansas Insurance Department
Consumer Services Division
Third and Cross Streets
Little Rock, AR 72201
(501) 371-2640

California

Department of Corporations
980 9th Street, Suite #500
Sacramento, CA 95814-3860
(916) 445-7205

Consumer Services Unit
(800) 400-0815

Colorado

Division of Insurance
1560 Broadway, Suite #850
Denver, CO 80202
(303) 894-7499

Consumer Affairs Division
(800) 930-3745

Connecticut

Insurance Department
P.O. Box 816
Hartford, CT 06142-0816
(860) 297-3900

Consumer Affairs Division
(800) 203-3447

Delaware

Department of Insurance
841 Silver Lake Boulevard
Dover, DE 19904
(302) 739-4251

Consumer Affairs and Investigations Division
(800) 282-8611

Florida

Department of Insurance
200 East Gaines Street
Tallahassee, FL 32399-0300
(850) 922-3100

Insurance Consumer Helpline
(800) 342-2762

Georgia

Commissioner of Insurance
2 Martin Luther King, Jr. Drive
West Tower, Suite # 704
Atlanta, GA 30334
(404) 656-2070

Consumer Services
(800) 656-2298

Hawaii

Insurance Division
250 S. King Street, 5th Floor
Honolulu, HI 96813
(808) 586-2790

Consumer Complaints
(808) 974-4000 ext. 62790 (from island of Hawaii)

Otherwise (808) 586-2790

Idaho

Department of Insurance
700 W. State Street, 3rd Floor
P.O. Box 83720
Boise, ID 83720-0043
(208) 334-4320

Consumer Affairs Division
(800) 721-3272

Illinois

Department of Insurance
320 W. Washington, 4th Floor
Springfield, IL 62767-0001
(217) 782-4515

Consumer Services
(217) 782-4515 or (312) 814-2427

Indiana

Department of Insurance
311 W. Washington Street
Suite #300
Indianapolis, IN 46204-2787
(317) 232-2395

Consumer Services
(800) 622-4461

Iowa

Insurance Division
330 Maple Street
Des Moines, IA 50319-0065
(515) 281-5705 or (515) 281-4241

Kansas

Insurance Department
420 SW 9th Street
Topeka, KS 66612
(785) 296-7850

Consumer Assistance Hotline
(800) 432-2484

Kentucky

Department of Insurance
Attn: Consumer Protection
P.O. Box 517
Frankfort, KY 40602-0517
(502) 564-6034

Consumer protection and Education Division
(800) 595-6053

Louisiana

Department of Insurance
P.O. Box 94214
Baton Rouge, LA 70804-9214
(225) 342-5900

Consumer Complaints
(800) 259-5300

Maine

Bureau of Insurance
Life and Health Division
#34 State House Maine
Augusta, ME 04333-0034
(207) 624-8475

Consumer Complaints
(800) 300-5000

Maryland

Insurance Administration
525 St. Paul Place
Baltimore, MD 21202-2272
(410) 468-2090

Consumer Complaints
(800) 492-6116 ext. 2244

Massachusetts

Division of Insurance
Consumer Service Section
470 Atlantic Ave.
Boston, MA 02210-2223
(617) 521-7794

Consumer Services Section
(617) 521-7777

Michigan

Insurance Bureau
P.O. Box 30220
Lansing, MI 48909-7720
(517) 373-9273

Consumer Complaints
(517) 373-0240

Minnesota

Department of Commerce
133 east 7th Street
St. Paul, MN 55101
Attention: Enforcement Division
(651) 296-2488

Department of Health
Health Policy & Systems
Compliance Division
Managed Care Section
(651) 282-5600

Department of Commerce
(800) 657-3602

Department of Health
Managed Care Systems Information
(800) 657-3916

Mississippi

Insurance Department
Consumer Services Division
P.O. Box 79
Jackson, MS 39205
(601) 359-3579

Consumer Services Division
(800) 562-2957

Missouri

Department of Insurance
P.O. Box 690
Jefferson City, MO 65102-0690
(573) 751-2640

Department of Insurance
Wainwright Building, Suite 229
111 N.7th Street
St. Louis, MO 63101
(314) 340-6830

Department of Insurance
State Office Building, Room 512
615 E. 13th Street
Kansas City, MO 64106-2829
(816) 889-2381

Montana

Consumer Complaints Division
P.O. Box 4009
Helena, MT 59604-4009
(406) 444-2040

Policy Holder Services
Consumer Complaints
(800) 332-6148

Nebraska

Department of Insurance
Terminal Building
941 O Street, Suite 400
Lincoln, NE 69508-3690
(402) 471-2201

Consumer Affairs Division
Toll free: (877) 564-7323

Nevada

Department of Business and Industry
Division of Insurance
1665 Hot Springs Road, Suite 152
Carson City, NV 89706
(775) 687-4270

Consumer Services
(800) 992-0900 or (888) 872-3234

New Hampshire

Insurance Department
56 Old Suncook Road
Concord, NH 03301-5151
(603) 271-2261

Consumer Assistance
(800) 852-3416

New Jersey

Division of Insurance
Enforcement and Consumer Complaints
P.O. Box 329
Trenton, NJ 08625-0329
(609) 292-5316

Department of Health and Senior Services
Office of Managed Care
P.O. Box 360
Trenton, NJ 08625-0360
(609) 588-2611

Division of Insurance
(800) 446-7467 (In New Jersey)

New Mexico

Public Relations Commission
Consumer Division
P.O. Box 1269
Santa Fe, NM 87504-1269
(505) 827-4592

Consumer Division
(800) 947-4722

New York

Consumer Services Bureau
NYS Insurance Department
Agency Bldg. 1-ESP
Albany, NY 12257
(518) 474-6600

Consumer Services Bureau
NYS Insurance Department
25 Beaver Street
New York, NY 10004-2319
(212) 480-6400

Consumer Services Bureau
NYS Insurance Department
65 Court Street-#7
Buffalo, NY 14202
(716) 847-7618

Consumer Services Bureau
(800) 342-3736 (All of New York)

North Carolina

Department of Insurance
P.O. Box 26387
Raleigh, NC 27611
(919) 733-7343

Consumer Services
(800) 546-5664

North Dakota

Department of Insurance
600 E. Boulevard, Department #401
Bismarck, ND 58505-0320
(701) 328-2440 or 800-247-0560

Oklahoma

Insurance Department
P.O. Box 53408
3814 N. Santa Fe
Oklahoma City, OK 73152-3408
(405) 521-28289

Customer Assistance
(800) 522-0071

Department of Health
HMO Complaint Assistance Line
(800) 811-4552

Ohio

Department of Insurance
2100 Stella Ct.
Columbus, OH 43215-1067
(614) 644-2658

Consumer Service Division
(800) 686-1526

Oregon

Department of Consumer and Business Services
Insurance Division
Consumer Protection Section
350 Winter St. NE, Room 440-2
Salem, OR 97310-0765
(503) 947-7980

Consumer Protection Division
(503) 947-7984

Pennsylvania

Bureau of Managed Care
Department of Health
P.O. Box 90
Health and Welfare Building
Harrisburg, PA 17108
(717) 787-5193

Bureau of Managed Care Division
(888) 466-2787

Rhode Island

Department of Health
Division of Health Services Regulation
Office of Managed Care Regulation
3 Capitol Hill, Room 410
Providence, RI 02908
(401) 222-6015

South Carolina

Department of Insurance
1612 Marion Street
P.O. Box 100105
Columbia, SC 29202
(803) 737-6150

Consumer Services
(800) 768-3467

South Dakota

Division of Insurance
118 West Capitol
Pierre, SD 57501
(605) 773-3563

Tennessee

Department of Commerce and Insurance
500 James Robertson Parkway
Nashville, TN 37243-0574
(615) 741-2218

Consumer Services
(800) 342-4029

Texas

Department of Insurance
Consumer Protection Program (111-1A)
P.O. Box 149091
Austin, TX 78714-9091
(512) 305-7211

Consumer Complaints
(800) 599-7467

Consumer Help Line
(800) 252-3439

Information Line for denials deemed not "medically necessary"
(888) 834-2476
(512) 322-3400 (in Austin)

Utah

Insurance Department
Consumer Service Division
State Office Building-Room 3110
Salt Lake City, UT 84114
(801) 538-3805

Consumer Service Division
(800) 439-3805

Vermont

Department of Banking, Insurance, Securities and Health Care Administration
VHCA Office
89 Main St. Drawer 20
Montpelier, VT 05620-3601
(802) 631-7788

Virginia

Bureau of Insurance
P.O. Box 1157
Richmond, VA 23218
(804) 371-9206

Consumer Services
(800) 552-7945

Washington

Insurance Commissioner
Consumer Advocacy and Outreach
P.O. Box 40256
Olympia, WA 98504-0256
(360) 753-3613

Consumer Advocacy Division
(800) 562-6900

Statewide Health Insurance Hotline
(800) 397-4422

West Virginia

Insurance Commission
Consumer Services Division
P.O. Box 50540
1124 Smith Street
Charleston, WV 25305-0540
Consumer Services Division
(800) 642-9004

Wisconsin

Office of the Commissioner of Insurance
Information and Complaints Section
P.O. Box 7873
Madison, WI 53707-7873
(608) 266-3585

Consumer Complaints
(800) 236-8517

Wyoming

Insurance Department
122 W. 25th Street
Herschler Bldg., 3rd Floor East
Cheyenne, WY 82002
(307) 777-7401

Consumer Assistance
(800) 438-5768

Note: This information was kindly provided by *Patients are Powerful.* Their web site is www.patientsarepowerful.org and their telephone number is (916) 652-2293.

HELPFUL WEB SITES

The Managed Care Patient Advocate
www.comed.com/empower
(215) 592-1363

National Committee for Quality Assurance
www.ncga.org
(800) 839-6487
Keep records regarding insurance plans

American Medical Association
www.ama-assn.org
(312) 464-5000

American Dental Association
www.ada.org
(312) 440-2500

Vial of Life
www.mypreciouskid.com/com/vial2.html
(503) 324-7323

Partnership for Caring
www.partnershipforcaring.org
Has Advanced Directive Forms that can be downloaded.
(800) 989-9455

California Department of Corporations
www.corp.ca.gov
(800) 248-2341 or (800) 400-0815

American Board of Medical Specialists

www.abms.org

(866) 275-2267

American Academy of Pediatrics

www.aap.org

(888) 227-1770

Medicare

www.medicare.gov

(800) 633-4227

Medic Alert

www.medicalert.org

(800) 344-3226

Association of Ambulatory Health Care

www.aaahc.org

Joint Commission on Accreditation of Healthcare Organizations

www.jcaho.org

American Bar Association

www.abanet.org

(312) 988-5000

Family Voices

www.ichp.ufl.edu/Family Voices

(505) 867-2368

Families USA

www.familiesusa.org

(202) 626-3030

National Protection and Advocacy
www.protectionandadvocacy.com
(800) 776-5746

Fractured Atlas
www.fracturedatlas.org
A nonprofit arts organization that provides low cost health coverage

Healthy New York
www.ins,state.ny.us/healthy.html
(866) 432-5849
Provides health insurance for low-income working people

Health Insurance Association of America
www.hiaa.org

Veterans Benefits
www.va.gov

Center for Medicare Advocacy
www.mecareadovcacy.org

Center for Health Dispute Resolution
www.healthappeal.com

The Medicine Program
www.themedicineprogram.com
Helps patients who can not afford prescriptions

Health Finder
www.healthfinder.gov

Health Gate
www.healthgte.com

Patients Are Powerful

www.patientsarepowerful.org

Center for Patient Advocacy

www.patientadvocacy.org

(800) 646-7444

Patients Who Care

www.patients.org

(800) 800-5154

Citizens Council on Health Care

www.cchc-mn/.org

(651) 646-8935

Omni Medical Search

www.omnimedicalsearch.com

Health Insurance Rate Comparison

www.ehealthinsurance.com

International Health

www.internationalsos.com

Medical Matrix

www.medmatrix.org

WebMD

www.webmd.com

Medscape

www.medscape.com

Intelihealth

www.intelihealth.com

Health A to Z

www.healthatoz.com

Mayo Clinic Health

www.mayohealth.org

Attention Deficit Hyperactivity Disorder

www.healing-arts.org/children/ADHD

Pediatric Asthma

www.peiatric-asthma.org

Immunizations

www.immunizationinfo.org

Health Finder

www.healthconnect.com

Patient Advocate

www.patientadvocate.org

Foundation for Taxpayer and Consumer Rights

www.consumerwathcdog.org

LifeFone

Personal response services

www.lifeone.com

American Women's Medical Association

www.amwa-doc.org

Magic Search Words for Better Health

www.MagicSearchWords.com

Appealing Insurance Medical Claims

www.kff.org/consumerguide

Helps Purchase Medicine

www.themedicineprogram.com

Kids Together, Inc.

Information and Resources for Children with Disabilities.

www.kidstogether.org

Patient Access, Inc.

Patient Advocacy

www.home.patientaccess.com/pac

Depression and Bipolar Support Alliance

www.DBSAlliance.org

(800) 826-3632

National Committee for Quality Assurance

www.ncqa.org

(800) 839-6478

Center for Children with Chronic Illness and Disability

www.peds.umn.edu

(612) 626-2134

Medicare Rights Center

www.medicarerights.org

Homecare Online

www.nahc.org

Visiting Nurse Association of America

www.vnaa.org

Mayo Clinic

www.mayo.edu

American Cancer Society

www.cancer.org

Health Answers

www.healthanswers.com

American Heart Association

www.americanheart.org

Arthritis Foundation

www.arthritis.org

American Stroke Association

www.americanheart.org/Stroke

National Organization of Rare Diseases

www.NORD-RDB.com

(800) 999-NORD

Muscular Dystrophy Family Foundation

www.mdff.org

(800) 544-1213

Medline Plus

www.nlm.nih.gov/medlineplus

Federal Drug Administration

www.fda.gov

www.fda.gov/buyonlineguide

www.fda.gov/medwatch

www.fda.gov/importeddrugs

www.fda.gov/cder/ogd

National Institutes of Health

www.nih.gov/health

Centers for Disease Control

www.cdc.gov

National Eye Institute

www.nei.nih.gov

National Institute of Mental Health

www.nimh.nih.gov

National Heart, Lung, and Blood Institute

www.nhlbi.nih.gov

National Institute of Diabetes and Digestive and Kidney Diseases

www.niddk.nih.gov

National Institute of Deafness and Communication Disorders

www.nih.gov/nidcd

National Institute of Neurological Disorders and Stroke

www.ninds.nih.gov

National Cancer Institute

www.nci.nih.gov

National Institute of Arthritis and Musculoskeletal and Skin Diseases

www.niams.nih/gov

National Institute of Allergy and Infectious Diseases

www.niaid.nih.gov

Comparing Hospitals

www.hospitalcompare.hhs.gov

Drug Reports

www.crbestbuydrugs.org/drugreports.html

Health Information

http://healthcarechoices.org

http://www.healthgrades.com

www.quackwatch.com

National Women's Health Information Center

www.4women.gov

American Hospice Foundation

www.americanhospice.org

(202) 223-0204

American Center for Assisted Living

www.ncal.org

(202) 842-4444

Veteran's Health Administration

www.va.gov

(877) 222-8387

National Association of Boards of Pharmacy

www.nabp.info

www.vipps.info

To find Internet suppliers meeting federal regulations.

STATE HIGH-RISK INSURANCE NUMBERS

Alabama
Alabama Health Insurance Plan
(800) 513-1384 or (334) 353-8924

Alaska
Alaska Comprehensive Health Insurance Association
(800) 467-8724 or (907) 269-7900

Arkansas
Arkansas Comprehensive Health Insurance Plan
(501) 278-2979

California
California Managed Risk Medical Insurance Program
(800) 289--6574 or (916) 324-4695

Colorado
Colorado Uninsurable Health Insurance Plan
(303) 863-1960

Connecticut
Connecticut Health Insurance Association
(800) 842-0004

Florida (not open for new enrollees)
Florida Comprehensive Health Insurance Plan
(850) 309-1200

Idaho
Department of Insurance
(202) 334-4250

Illinois
Illinois Comprehensive Health Insurance Plan
(800) 367-6410 or (217) 782-6333

Indiana
Indiana Comprehensive Health Insurance Association
(800) 552-7921 or (317) 614-2000

Iowa
Iowa Comprehensive Health Association
(800) 877-5156

Kansas
Kansas Uninsurable Health Insurance Plan
(800) 290-1366 or (316) 792-1779

Kentucky
Kentucky Access
(866) 405-6145

Louisiana
Louisiana Health Insurance Association
(800) 736-0947 or (504) 926-6245

Maryland
Maryland Health Insurance Plan
(866) 780-7105 or (410) 576-2055

Minnesota
Minnesota Comprehensive Health Association
(952) 593-9609

Mississippi
Mississippi Comprehensive Health Insurance Risk Pool
(601) 362-0799

Missouri
Missouri Health Insurance Pool
Northwest Missouri: (800) 645-8346
Remainder of state: (800) 843-6447

Montana
Montana Comprehensive Health Insurance Association
(406) 444-8200

Nebraska
Nebraska Comprehensive Health Association
(402) 343-3337

New Hampshire
New Hampshire Health Plan
(800) 578-3272

New Mexico
New Mexico Comprehensive Health Insurance Pool
(505) 271-4399

North Dakota

Comprehensive Health Association of North Dakota

(800) 737-0016 or (701) 282-1235

Oklahoma

Oklahoma Health Insurance High Risk Pool

(800) 255-6065 or (913) 362-0040

Oregon

Oregon Medical Insurance Pool

(503) 373-1692

South Carolina

South Carolina Health Insurance Pool

(803) 788-0222

South Dakota

South Dakota Risk Pool

(800) 831-0785

Tennessee

TennCare Program

(615) 741-8642

Texas

Texas Health Insurance Risk Pool

(888) 398-3927 or (512) 441-7665

Utah

Utah Comprehensive Health Insurance Pool

(866) 880-8494 or (801) 333-5573

Washington

Washington State Health Insurance Pool

(800) 877-5187 or (360) 407-0380

Wisconsin

Wisconsin Health Insurance Risk Sharing Plan

(608) 264-7733

Wyoming

Wyoming Health Insurance Pool

(307) 634-1393

BIBLIOGRAPHY

Anders, George. *Health Against Wealth: HMOs and the Breakdown of Medical Trust* .New York: Houghton Mifflin, 1996.

Cooperman, Tod, William Obermeyer and Denise Webb. *Guide to Buying Vitamins and Supplements.* ConsumerLab, 2003.

Court, Jamie and Smith, Francis. *Making a Killing: HMOs and the Threat to Your Health.* Monroe, ME: Common Courage Press, 1999.

Eban, Katherine. *Dangerous Doses.* New York: HarperBooks, 2005.

Einteen, Robert. *Health Insurance: How to Get It, Keep It or Improve What You've Got.* New York: Demos Vermande, 1996.

Graedon, Joe and Theresa Graedon. *The People's Guide to Deadly Drug Interaction.* New York: St. Martin's Press, 1995.

Jablonski, Stanley. *Dictionary of Medical Acronyms and Abbreviations.* Philadelphia, Pa: Hauley & Belfus, Inc. 2001.

LeBow, Robert H. *Health Care Meltdown.* Chambersburg, PA: Alan C.Hood & Co. 2003.

PDR for Herbal Medicines. Montvale, NJ. Thomson Healthcare, Inc. 2004.

Shernoff, William. *Fight Back and Win, How to Get Your HMO to Pay Up.,* Greenwich, CT: Board Room Books, 1999. (1-203-625-5900)

Thompson, Charlotte. *Raising a Child with a Neuromuscular Disorder*. New York, NY: Oxford University Press, 2000.

Thompson, Charlotte. *Raising a Handicapped Child.* New York, NY: Oxford University Press, 1999.